Essential Oils: The Step-by-Step Guide to Essential Oils from A-Z for Weight Loss, Stress Relief and Aromatherapy

By Malik Johnson

Copyright 2015 by WE CANT BE BEAT LLC

Published by WE CANT BE BEAT LLC

krob817@yahoo.com

Table of Contents

Introduction

The Healing Power of Aromatherapy: The Knowledge of Ancient Civilizations

Aromatherapy is the ancient therapeutic practice of using pure plant-derived essential oils to heal, protect and rejuvenate the body and mind. As the name suggests, aroma or scent plays a very important role in the balancing and restorative techniques of aromatherapy. Fragrant essential oils derived from flowers and plants are used to positively affect the physical and mental health because they contain all of the active benefits of the plants they are sourced from, in much higher amounts. These benefits are so deeply concentrated within these oils that they work quickly and effectively, making aromatherapy one of the most healing methods of treatment for a wide variety of conditions.

However, when most people think of healing, they immediately link it to using medicine. Anything outside of the realm of modern prescription drugs is considered an "alternative" or "unproven" therapy that has little chance of actually working. Society tends to think this way because the modern world is completely addicted to the chemical medications that doctors freely prescribe. We've become convinced that nature has no healing power and no place in real hospitals and clinics and we have come to believe that we can only trust treatment options that come from a pharmaceutical lab, not from the natural world. I'm here to tell you that this idea is simply not true. The fact is, our bodies are natural and they instinctively respond best to the treatments provided by the natural world, over the chemical – loaded, toxic medications of today. Long before the advent of conventional medicine, the flowers and plants around us were our primary (and highly beneficial!) source of health. Sadly, while ancient civilizations before us relied heavily on plants for healing, we have forgotten this powerful secret

From Ancient Egypt, India and China, to Renaissance Europe, humans have successfully used the ancient healing powers of aromatherapy for many thousands of years. Long before the modern prescription drugs of today, we knew how to extract, concentrate and use the amazing natural properties of plants to heal, cleanse, detoxify and protect our bodies and soothe our minds. These were not simply home remedies without scientific proof. In fact, these paths to healing have stood the test of time and are now even being recognized by top researchers and scientists around the world, as potent and viable health promoting options.

So if essential oils and aromatherapy worked so well in the past, why aren't they more widely used today?

Well, the truth is, millions of people are becoming very interested in learning how to use these all-natural curatives to heal issues that modern medicine and doctors just can't seem to figure out. Because the pills, tablets and treatments of today aren't able to solve many of the medical mysteries and difficult to treat diseases we are increasingly seeing, essential oils and aromatherapy are quickly regaining their former popularity and have become important weapons in the war against modern-day diseases. Many people have had to scour the internet and look for knowledge in books such as this one to discover the right and beneficial ways to use these ancient healing tools because quite frankly, essential oils and aromatherapy were forgotten for many years. People lost their link to the ancient and proven benefits of natural products and began to rely only on prescription medications. But today, there is a huge resurgence of interest in using these tools for two very simple reasons: Essential oils and aromatherapy work very well as gentle, effective additional healing tools AND they are much less expensive than most conventional treatments out there today.

On the other hand, science and modern-day scientists are also firmly convinced that only synthetic, "technologically advanced" medicines really work. So all of these factors have worked together to keep most people in the dark about the benefits of essential oils and aromatherapy. Aromatherapy was very widely used and known as a proven therapy for a range of illnesses and disorders until the 19th century. New medical techniques in this period caused scientists and doctors alike to believe that we no longer needed nature's bounty because we had learned how to replicate the healing properties of plants in a laboratory. But we human beings are living creatures and it's only logical that our natural systems respond best to natural treatments. And think about this: If plants and their properties are so powerful and useful to human health that pharmaceutical companies make copies of them in labs for medicinal uses, why don't we also use the originals that nature provided?

 And that's where aromatherapy comes in. When done properly and with all of the knowledge provided in this book, aromatherapy is one of the single most powerful healers in the world. It is all about harnessing natural cures to alleviate, heal and prevent every kind of health problem. Because of this, it is increasingly sought after by millions of people who are tired of poisoning their bodies and minds with toxic, modern, chemically produced pills and who want an option that is strong enough to truly treat them but is also so natural that it won't harm them like harsh meds do.

While many diseases do benefit from the use of conventional medications and you should never limit yourself to only one healing method over another, essential oils and aromatherapy can often add an intensely beneficial second dimension to any treatment plan you are already following. This is why all pharmaceutical companies have based their most successful medications, from aspirin to valium, on the blueprint of nature.

Ancient cultures also used essential oils as natural cleaning and anti-bacterial, anti-microbial and anti-fungal products and new research shows that they were right to do so. In fact, when scientists studied essential oils, they found that many of them were able to effectively battle deadly bacteria and super-bug strains. In some cases, these natural essential oils have been found to be even more effective than the extra-strength modern cleaners and bleaches we all rely on so heavily these days.

As you can see, ancient people knew very well what we are just beginning to remember: that despite all of the huge medical leaps of modern times, nature's pharmacopeia is absolutely packed with amazing remedies and cures for every human ailment and disorder.

You may be wondering: **What Can Essential Oils and Aromatherapy Do for Me?**

The answer to that is, quite simply everything. Anything that modern, conventional medicine can do for your health, fitness and well-being, aromatherapy can also do, and can often do it in a better, safer and more truly effective way! Using vibrant plant components in diffusions, inhalations, topical applications, baths and the healing touch of massage, aromatherapy targets and eliminates everything from every day pains to serious, life-threatening diseases.

Whether it is treating anxiety and depression, promoting weight loss, cooling inflammation, improving concentration, preventing infectious and non-communicable diseases or sharpening the brain, there is an aromatherapy method and an amazing essential oil that can help your to achieve all of these goals. Perhaps the very best part about this aromatherapy guide is that gives you all of the safety information and techniques you need to take your own healing into your own hands.

What's In This Book?

Whatever your health concern may be, this A-Z guide is packed with alphabetically categorized essential oils and aromatherapy methods to help you resolve any illness or disorder, in a natural yet powerful way. It includes in-depth explanations of the specific properties of each essential oil, which issues and conditions it works to heal and how best to use it. I've chosen the ultimate essential oils for almost every letter of the alphabet and made sure that once you've read the chapter, you will be totally equipped with the knowledge you need to, in order to use that oil properly. This book also contains critical safety information, so that you can get all of the positives out of your oils, without having to worry about making a potentially risky decision. Because essential oils are extremely powerful, it is absolutely vital that you know the correct ways to use them, to avoid placing yourself and your loved ones in harm's way.

Included at the very end of this book is a bonus index of the most powerfully healing, energizing and rebalancing blends that you can easily whip up, to access amazing health, weight loss and brain-boosting rewards in moments!

If you're looking for genuine restoration, rejuvenation and revitalization, all you have to do is turn the page and get blending, diffusing and inhaling. I guarantee that once you experience the intense relief that essential oils provide, you' will never want to be without a cupboard full of these natural cure-alls again. Are you ready for aromatherapy to restore your health, sharpen your mind and completely transform your life? Great, let's get started!

Chapter 1:

A.

Angelica Root Essential Oil:

Angelica root essential oil is a very aromatic oil extracted from the angelica root plant. It produces a scent that is at once green and herb-like as well as spiced and peppery. When used in aromatherapy, this oil offers several useful benefits to the health, including depurative, diuretic and relaxing effects.

It's loaded with active constituents like alpha pinene, beta pinene, camphene, alpha phellandrene, beta phellandrene, bornyl acetate, limonene and sabinene, making it one of the most dynamic and useful natural substances used in aromatherapy. Let's look at some of the very best uses for this rich and healing essential oil:

For its Depurative Abilities:

Angelica oil is a great depurative or blood purifying substance. This essential oil has long been widely used to draw out and eliminate waste products, harmful toxins and other unwanted buildup from the body through various means. It is extremely effective at supporting the body's own natural detoxification pathways, by offering enhanced renal and sweat-based elimination, so add this oil to your regimen of massages and inhalations, in order to promote a complete, total body detox.

For its Diuretic Properties:

This oil is also a famous diuretic, often used for its ability to stimulate urination. This property is important because as the body begins to frequently pass urine, it also gets rid of many harmful toxins and pollutants backed up inside the blood and organs, such as excessive salt, uric acid, harmful fats and large amounts of unused bile. In this way, the oil prevents and treats conditions like rheumatism, gout, arthritis and kidney stress, by aiding in the timely removal of unwanted byproducts and waste.

As high percentages of fat can also be ushered out through regular urination and blood pressure is also significantly lowered in the process, the diuretic properties of angelica root oil are often used to achieve and maintain weight loss and treat hypertension.

For its Diaphoretic Qualities:

Yet another very useful property of angelica root oil is its ability to promote heavy sweating. Now, this may not seem like a particularly helpful effect in the context of day-to-day living but when we want to achieve serious detoxification, it is absolutely vital.

That's because sweating is your body's natural process for eliminating dangerous toxic waste. Every time you sweat, your body is busily offloading unnecessary uric acids, fats, bile and even excessive sebum. If these things are allowed to remain within the body, they can cause a dangerous backlog of waste products and trigger everything from inflammation to major illnesses. Using angelica root oil in massages, soaks and inhalations allows the body to sweat fully leading to wonderful benefits such as a purified body, lowered inflammation and a better potassium ratio within the blood, which is linked to a decrease in blood pressure. Sweating, as many who use saunas for detox know, can also promote a faster metabolism and create the right conditions for weight loss!

For its Liver Protectant Effects:

Adding to angelica root oil's long list of purifying qualities is its ability to cleanse, protect and even heal the liver. Not only does this oil remove harmful waste products that could inflame and damage the liver, it also triggers beneficial secretions that maintain proper liver function. Angelica root oil also works in a targeted manner to fight off and heal any infections within the liver, preventing swelling, scarring and failure within this sensitive organ.

For its Nerve-Healing Properties:

If you need a natural nerve healer and tonic, look no further than this essential oil. It's famous for its ability to strengthen and protect the nerves from a variety of disorders and improve the function of the entire nervous system. Angelica root oil is unique in that, it contains both deeply relaxing and highly stimulating components. The result is that this oil can be used to stimulate nerve activity and blood circulation, helping the nerves to receive necessary blood, while also imparting a sense of calm and carefully balancing nerve function, to prevent any hyperactivity.

Aromatherapy:

There are several ways to access angelica root essential oil's cleansing, purifying, diuretic and nerve-health boosting benefits. Try an immersion treatment by adding 8-10 drops of pure angelica root oil to a warm bath, or use 3-4 drops to infuse the air of a sauna. As you soak in the tub or sit in the sauna, make a point of inhaling the fragrant air deep into your lungs several times. This will draw even more of the oil's benefits into the body and allow its properties to work internally. For relaxation, during the day, place 2 drops of angelica oil diluted in a teaspoon and a half of coconut oil on each wrist and rub together before smelling. In the evenings, induce a peaceful sensation and set the stage for great sleep by placing 2-3 drops of the oil on your pillow and bed sheets. Inhaling the scent as you sleep will deepen and improve the quality of your night's rest. For a full body massage that will aid in detoxification, blend 4-5 drops of angelica oil in 2 tablespoons of almond oil and work thoroughly into the skin. Allow this oil to sit on the skin for at least an hour before washing off thoroughly in warm water. The oil will work to pull up impurities and washing vigorously will help to eliminate them from the body.

Precautions to Remember:

Essential oils contain all of the active components of the plants they are expressed or distilled from, but they contain these components in an extremely concentrated form. Therefore, it's very important not to use these oils in large doses or with excessive frequency. Before applying angelica root oil topically, always dilute it with a suitable carrier oil, such as olive, jojoba, coconut or almond oil. 3-4 drops of angelic root oil should be blended with 1-2 tablespoons of your chosen carrier oil, before being applied to the skin. Angelica root oil can cause photosensitivity, if skin that has been treated with it is exposed to direct sunlight within 24 hours of treatment. Because the sweet scent tends to attract insects, this oil should not be used outdoors.

I recommend that those who are pregnant, nursing or are diabetic should avoid this oil and that medical advice should be sought before using it on young children, as it is very powerful. If inhaled in excess, it may contribute to nervousness and hyperactivity.

Chapter 2:

A.

Bay Essential Oil:

Whether you use it in topical applications or inhale its scent through diffusers and steam inhalation, bay essential oil offers a wide variety of wonderful effects. As an anti-inflammatory, a purgative and even an anti-depressant, this oil has become famous for its intensely rejuvenating properties. You can use bay oil in the following ways:

For its Anti-Inflammatory Effects:

One of bay oil's most valuable qualities is its inflammation-fighting ability. Because this oil is expressed from bay leaves, it is rich in the same amazing components, including a special phytonutrient called parthenolide.

Parthenolide has been shown to rapidly decrease inflammation when bay oil is used topically on aching muscles, painful bones and swollen arthritic joints. This oil can also cool inflammatory conditions of the skin and the scalp through topical application and when inhaled in a diffused form, it works to soothe an inflamed or irritated respiratory system.

Digestive Health:

Bay oil has traditionally been used as a primarily digestive treatment. The scent has an almost immediate and very marked effect on the digestive system's functions. Bay oil can trigger diuretic effects, drawing toxins out of the body through urination. It is also an emetic, allowing the stomach to empty itself of potentially harmful substances quickly. These two properties make this oil a perfect antidote to the painful symptoms of Celiac disease. Bay essential oil can also be used in stomach rubs and steam inhalations, to calm IBS, reduce stomach spasms and allow for improved gastrointestinal functions.

For Prevention and Management of Diabetes:

Bay oil use has been linked to balancing of blood sugar levels and enhanced performance of insulin receptors, leading to a decreased risk of developing diabetes. The oil has also been shown to improve the health of those with preexisting diabetes.

For Depression and Anxiety:

Bay oil is full of linalool, a natural but very effective anxiety reliever. This substance works to dramatically decrease levels of stress hormone cortisol in the blood stream, resulting in a calmer, happier and clearer state of mind.

Aromatherapy:

Heal systemic inflammation by applying a blend of 3 drops of bay oil in an ounce of coconut oil to the chest, back and stomach area. Banish insomnia by diffusing 3-5 drops of pure bay oil throughout your bedroom half an hour before going to sleep. Get rid of anxiety and depression by massaging your body and temples with a blend of 4 drops of bay oil in a tablespoon of almond oil. Ease scalp pain and ward off dandruff by placing 1-2 drops of bay oil in your favorite shampoo and allowing the mixture to sit on the scalp for at least 10 minutes, before rinsing.

It is also crucial to remember that bay oil, as well as bay rum and the fruit of the Bay tree, possesses toxic properties and should not be ingested

Precautions to Remember:
Although certain essential oils are safe for consumption, bay oil is highly toxic and should never be taken internally. Avoid skin sensitization by always diluting this oil in a carrier such as olive or coconut oil. Pregnant and nursing women as well as anyone with a health condition should consult a doctor before use. This oil should not be used on young children unless otherwise advised by a medical professional.
Make sure that you only use pure bay oil from the laurel tree, otherwise known *Laurus nobilis*, to reap

all of the benefits listed above. Other types of "bay oil" are not authentic and can result in toxicity, allergies and contact dermatitis.

Chapter 3:

C.

Cinnamon Oil:

For Weight Loss:

Cinnamon oil is one of the most powerful essential oils you can use to support your weight loss plan. It has a proven blood glucose level balancing and regulating effect and has also shown its effectiveness at regulating your body's glucose tolerance factor. We know that controlling your blood glucose levels and your glucose tolerance are key parts of losing weight and keeping it off, so this makes cinnamon essential oil an excellent tool for long term weight loss.

When you use cinnamon oil, two things begin to happen in your body almost immediately. One is, as mentioned, your blood sugar levels stabilize, leading to more efficient fat-burning. The other is that you find you're no longer experiencing the usual desperate cravings for carbohydrate and sugar – loaded foods that are the biggest reason for failed diets. Instead, you begin to eat only when you're actually hungry and the need for those calorie-packed snacks goes away.

For Stress Relief:

Cinnamon essential oil is known to have an anti-depressive and relaxing effect. It works particularly well for those who are suffering from SAD (seasonal affective disorder) and who tend to feel low and anxious during the colder winter months. Cinnamon oil contains eugenol, which is highly effective at soothing and relaxing the body and easing the strain that comes from immune disorders like fibromyalgia and rheumatic arthritis.

Aromatherapy:

The best way to use cinnamon essential oil to support your weight loss is to add 1-2 drops of it to an aromatherapy diffuser and inhale its scent in the morning. Cinnamon oil's ability to stabilize your blood sugar levels and eliminate your food cravings makes it a fantastic way to start your day off.

To gain relaxation, add just a few drops of cinnamon essential oil to your base oil for a deeply relaxing massage that will relieve your physical and mental stress. Just make sure that you do not add more than 2 drops of cinnamon oil per 0.16 ounces of base oil.

For Hair Growth:

Cinnamon essential oil also makes a great natural treatment for thinning hair or limp lifeless strands that just won't grow. Because cinnamon oil is a follicle stimulator, it penetrates deep into the scalp to improve blood flow to your hair follicles and provides the proper circulation that hair needs in order to grow. It has been proven to work in both male pattern balding and general thinning. Cinnamon oil is also loaded with important antioxidants that root out and destroy free radicals. This helps to eliminate all inflammation in the scalp area and means that hair can grow thickly and to its full potential. To get the benefits for yourself, first do a small patch test at the nape of your neck, or behind an ear, to make sure your delicate scalp area will not develop an allergic reaction to the oil. If after 48 hours the skin you tested has not developed redness, irritation or itchiness, dilute 2 drops of the cinnamon oil into natural base oil like jojoba and massage into the scalp. Focus on working the oil into areas where hair is thinning or you desire thicker growth. Regularly using this blend up to 3 times a week for several weeks in a row will help you to achieve the hair growth results you seek.

Precautions to Remember: Cinnamon oil is naturally high in cinnamaldehyde and eugenol and these two substances may sometimes cause skin and mucus membrane irritation, if applied directly and not properly diluted. Because of its ability to stimulate blood flow to the uterus, cinnamon essential oil should never be used in any form during pregnancy.

Clove Oil:

For Weight Loss: Cloves come from the medicinal evergreen tree's buds and are indigenous to the islands of Madagascar and Indonesia. Clove oil is an amazing anti-inflammatory essential oil. It has literally dozens of uses, from protecting the liver and fighting gum disease to clearing acne. Because of its inflammation-fighting powers, clove oil can also be used for weight loss. When your body is inflamed, your number one weight–controlling hormone leptin becomes less efficient and you end up gaining weight, even without increasing the amount of calories you eat. Taking clove oil internally can reduce inflammation levels in your body and help leptin to work properly, contributing to weight loss. Cloves oil is rich in compounds that speed up your metabolism and enhance fat-burning.

In addition, many people who experience unexplained weight gain are actually suffering from a candida infection. Candida infections can slow down the metabolism, cause bloating and swelling and result in pounds stubbornly piling up. The anti-fungal substances found in clove oil are proven candida killers, completely rooting out and destroying all fungal infections within the body and restoring a bloated, heavy body to its normal state.

For Stress Relief: If you're looking for an essential oil to soothe your frayed nerves and calm your stressed out mind and body, clove oil is a wonderful choice. In fact, it has such a relaxing effect on the nervous system that it can even be used as a mild sedative and sleep aid. Because clove oil is an anti-clotting agent and also lowers blood pressure, it provides a gently relaxing effect and can even help to reduce any muscular aches and back pains, making it easier for you to slip into deep, restful sleep.

For Coughs, Colds and Other Respiratory Complaints: To loosen and remove hard to dislodge mucus during a bad bout of the flu or a cold, try a clove oil steam inhalation. Fill a large bowl with hot water and blend in 2-3 drops of clove oil. Keep your face at least 12 inches away from the bowl, cover your head and the bowl with a large, clean cloth and make a tent. Breathe in deeply, pulling the scented steam deep into your nose and mouth. Each time you inhale this fragrant steam, you will be removing infected mucus from your respiratory system and breathing in anti-bacterial, anti-viral and anti-fungal steam. Additionally, you'll be drawing the anti-inflammatory and anti-stress properties of clove oil into your system.

Aromatherapy: Harness the powers of clove oil with an aromatherapy foot rub. To use clove oil for a foot rub, first prepare the area to receive the oil by soaking feet in a warm bath. Towel off and apply 2-3 drops of the clove oil, blended into one ounce of olive or coconut oil, to the feet. Massage the oil deeply into the skin, using firm circular motions and concentrating on the soles of the feet. Because feet contain important pressure points, the entire body will benefit from this massage as the clove oil affects these points.

Precautions to Remember: Three different types of clove oil can be produced from the evergreen tree. These are clove leaf oil, clove stem oil and clove bud oil. Clove bud oil is the favored by aromatherapists because it is the most active, beneficial and safe of the 3 types. When you select a clove essential oil, makes sure that you choose pure clove bud oil and that you always mix 2-3 drops of the oil into carrier oils such as olive, jojoba or coconut oil, before applying to skin. Diluting he oil means that you can access all of its benefits while avoiding any burns or irritation from direct skin contact. Because clove oil can result in photosensitivity, make sure that you keep areas that have come into contact with the oil out of direct sunlight. For safety, it is also recommended that you avoid using clove oil during pregnancy or nursing.

Chapter 4:

D.

Dill Seed Oil

For Weight Loss: While it offers many benefits, ranging from curing respiratory diseases to healing infections of all kinds, dill see oil's greatest powers are in its digestive properties. Because good digestion is the foundation of any effective weight loss plan, dill seed oil has been used since ancient times to treat obesity and to control weight levels. Dill seed oil works by strengthening and toning the gastric mucosa and the entire digestive system, providing major anti-inflammatory benefits and reducing the appetite. When all 3 properties are combined, you'll find that previously stubborn fat simply starts slipping off.

For Stress Relief: Dill seed oil acts as an inflammation cooler, making it a perfect cure for a stressed out, unhappy or nervous mind. Researchers have found that inflammatory conditions in the brain are often to blame for a large percentage of depression and anxiety cases. By calming the flames of cerebral inflammation with dill seed oil, you can restore and rebalance your brain while healing and preventing long term stress disorders.

For Nausea and Vomiting: When you can't seem to hold anything down and conventional medicine isn't easing that queasy feeling, try a whiff of dill seed oil. This oil's deeply anti-spasmodic and carminative properties help to ease the cramps and spasms of nausea and stabilize the stomach. Simply holding a small bottle of dill seed oil up to 5 inches away from your nose and breathing in can put an end to your suffering.

Aromatherapy: To use dill seed oil most effectively, it is best to take a 2 pronged approach. For weight loss and digestive benefits, add up to 3 drops of dill seed oil to an unscented, simple lotion or cream and massage your body daily with the blend. Pay special attention to rubbing the lotion into the skin covering your abdominal area, as this will concentrate the digestive healing powers of dill seed oil. At the same time, add 2 drops of dill seed oil to a clean, unscented aromatherapy pillow and breathe in the calming, sedative and anti –inflammatory scent of dill as you sleep. In the morning, you're sure to wake up feeling relaxed, more energetic and with fewer food cravings than usual.

Precautions to Remember: As with all essential oils, dilute dill seed oil fully before using directly on the face, mucus membranes or body and speak with your doctor before using this oil if pregnant.

Douglas Fir Oil:

For Anti-Viral Protection: The concentrated essential oil of Douglas fir pine trees has intensely anti-viral properties. If you are in need of a strong but safe and all-natural form of prevention during the dreaded flu season, try keeping a handkerchief soaked in up to 4 drops of the Douglas fir oil on hand at all times. When you are in uncomfortably close situations with others who may have the flu, you can breathe in the oil and instantly pull protection into your nose and mouth's vulnerable mucus membranes. Keep a small bottle of Douglas fir oil at your desk for a quick sniff that will help you stay healthy and cold-free all through the winter months.

For Anti-Bacterial Purposes: Douglas fir oil is also a known bacteria killer so if you need to freshen up a room or clean a surface that you fear may have a high bacterial load on it, simply add 5 drops of pure Douglas fir oil to a small amount of warm water and you have a potent anti-bacterial solution that you can use on countertops, door handles, gym equipment or any other area that requires anti-bacterial treatment.

For Stress Relief: Douglas fir oil, like all conifer tree essential oils, is a well-known remedy for an anxious state of mind. If you find yourself unable to relax or suffer from stress-based insomnia, try a soothing Douglas fir oil treatment at least half an hour before going to bed. Begin by running a warm bath. As the bath tub fills, add 5 drops of Douglas fir oil to the running water and allow the oil to disperse freely throughout the bath, before stepping in and soaking for a minimum of 20 minutes. Because Douglas fir oil also soothes tense muscles as it eases the mind, it is the perfect way to ensure a satisfying night of sleep.

Aromatherapy: To remove unwanted odors from a room or add anti-bacterial, anti-viral and anti-fungal protection to an area, apply 8 -10 drops of Douglas fir oil to a diffuser and allow the scent to circulate thoroughly. If you are in a room, try closing the doors and windows for 5 minutes to allow the scent to work before it is diluted by fresh air.

Precautions to Remember: If you are pregnant or nursing, please be sure to consult your doctor before using Douglas fir oil. Remember to dilute the oil in water or a safe carrier oil such as coconut, olive oil or jojoba oil before applying it directly to skin.

Chapter 5:

E.

Eucalyptus Oil:

For Weight Loss: Eucalyptus oil comes from the dried leaves of the eucalyptus tree, a native evergreen of Australia. Eucalyptus was traditionally used as a form of treatment against fevers, colds and body pains and today, it is both a proven fighter of inflammation and an infection-reducing agent. When it comes to weight loss, eucalyptus oil provides serious help to any diet plan by eliminating systemic inflammation. As the inflammatory conditions of your body cool down, your metabolism is better able to work at full speed, resulting in weight loss. Eucalyptus oil is also a fantastic anti-fungal option so if you suspect that a systemic fungal infection like candida is behind your bloating, swelling and weight gain, simply inhaling this powerful essential oil can reduce your body's fungal load quickly and easily.

Candida is also notorious for causing weight gain by increasing your cravings for sugary, carbohydrate-packed foods but eucalyptus oil's ability to control your body's hunger signals will help you to fight back against this fungal hunger. For quick craving control, lightly soak or spray a couple of cotton balls in eucalyptus oil and keep them in a Ziploc bag.

Whenever you feel hunger pangs coming on, simply reach for a cotton ball and inhale the scent. Your cravings will rapidly decrease, allowing you to make healthier meal choices instead of being controlled by candida.

For Pain Relief: Eucalyptus oil has proven analgesic, pain-relieving properties. Studies have found that putting diluted eucalyptus oil on areas where you feel pain results in effective reduction of aches and strains. You can also use eucalyptus oil as a form of pain prevention by thoroughly massaging the diluted oil into your muscles before a workout. The natural heat provided by the oil will help your muscles to warm up and will keep them safe from pulling or straining, no matter how hard you exercise.

For Stress Relief and Mental Rejuvenation: Whether you're overworked or you'd like to sharpen your brain's processes for a test or task, eucalyptus oil provides an excellent anxiety-reducing and mind renewing effect. It has an ability to ease stress, nervous tension and an exhausted mind by giving off a refreshing and cooling scent. Inhaling eucalyptus oil steam can increase blood flow to your brain, helping you to think more clearly, quickly and accurately. The next time you need to concentrate on an academic or work task, use a nebulizer to create eucalyptus oil steam and take several deep breaths at a range of 12 inches.

For Decongesting and Easier Breathing: If you suffer from seasonal allergies or have a constantly stuffy nose, eucalyptus oil can be your best friend. This essential oil's potent scent has the ability to open up blocked passageways in the nose, moth and chest areas, allowing you to breathe more comfortably. Once it opens up your nasal passages, you will also be able to remove any backed up mucus, so it is an important option for treating colds, flus and other respiratory illnesses like bronchitis. When you find it difficult to breath, reach for eucalyptus oil instead of an over-the-counter medication and you will be amazed by the instant results you get!

Aromatherapy:

Although diffusion and nebulizing are also great options for using eucalyptus oil, the most beneficial and healing method of use is in a warm full body soak. Draw a warm bath and allow 7 to 8 drops of eucalyptus oil to mix into the bath by placing the oil in the flowing water. Once the oil has spread, soak in the warm bath for up to half an hour. As you soak, focus on breathing the strong eucalyptus scent into your lungs.

If you have an area of particular soreness or strain, gently massage the eucalyptus oil-scented bath water into the skin covering the problem area. Because eucalyptus oil has a cooling effect, this bath should ideally be used in more temperate weather. During colder months, avoid stepping into an air-conditioned or extremely cool room immediately after a eucalyptus oil bath because the cooling effect may be doubled and result in an extremely low body temperature.

For Eliminating Mites and Insects:

If you have an insect or bed bug problem but you don't want to use harsh chemicals in the home, try nebulizing eucalyptus essential oil in the room. You can also douse the affected furniture or carpeting with a strong solution of eucalyptus oil and water. Add 8 to 10 drops of eucalyptus oil per cup of water, mix well, and spray the infested area with the blend. Many of the mites, ticks and insects you are dealing with will either die off or try to exit the area immediately. You can also use eucalyptus oil as a bug repellent in the garden. To get rid of ants, mites, white flies and other pests, simply mix 1o drops of eucalyptus oil with 1/3 cup of water. Pour the mixture into a spray bottle and shake well. Spray this mixture in the soil and mulch around plants that are being attacked by garden pests or directly onto the plants themselves and you will see a noticeable reduction in bugs, aphids and other garden hazards.

Precautions to Remember: Eucalyptus oil is one of the oldest and most widely used essential oils of all and is generally one of the safest oils as well. However, there are a few specific precautions to keep in mind when using it. I advise adults to use eucalyptus oil topically or in inhaled form. You should only use it orally if you are under medical supervision. Eucalyptus oil is highly concentrated so it may be too strong for the system and can even be toxic if taken in high enough doses.

Do not allow children to ingest eucalyptus oil and keep it out of their reach. Eucalyptus oil is normally quite safe to use on skin but it should not be used on children, as their skin is much more delicate than adult skin. Small pets may also become ill if they ingest this oil so keep them away from areas and rooms treated with a eucalyptus oil solution. Pregnant and nursing women should not use eucalyptus oil. If you use the oil on garden plants, make sure that your pets do not ingest any of the treated leaves, soil or mulch.

Chapter 6

F.

Fennel Oil:

For Detoxifying the Body: Fennel essential oil is a highly useful health tonic because it has both diuretic and laxative effects on the body. Using this oil while detoxing will help you to fully purge and remove any chemicals, metals and other toxins luring in your system. Because it stimulates the endocrine and exocrine glands in your body, fennel oil promotes the release of toxic materials through sweat and urine. Fennel oil promotes the expulsion of blood urea and uric acid. Add ½ a drop of fennel oil into a warm glass of water for an instant tonic and detoxifying effects. This will open up your system and allow any buildup to flow naturally out of you.

For Stress Relief and Mental Fatigue: As an all-over stimulant, fennel oil targets the brain and helps to revive and revitalize it. If you feel wiped out or too tired to think clearly, using fennel oil can clear away the brain fog and reenergize your thought process. The scent of fennel oil is also widely known as a great anti-depressant and can promote mood and mental stability, if sniffed a few times a day.

For Nausea: Fennel oil will stop nausea in its tracks with just one whiff. If you have lost your appetite or are experiencing stomach spasms, you can use the smell of fennel oil to get rid of these unpleasant effects. It can even promote proper secretions of stomach acid and mucus, keeping your entire digestive healthy and balanced. If your nausea is caused by an intestinal infection, you'll also benefit from fennel oil's vermifuge properties. Fennel oil is a powerful worm and parasite killer that can destroy spores before they grow into a major health problem.

Aromatherapy: Add on drop of fennel oil on to the palm of your hand rub both hands together and bring palms to your nose. Inhale deeply for revitalization. Add ½ a drop of fennel oil into a warm glass of water for an instant tonic and detoxifying effects.

Precautions to Remember: Do not use fennel oil if you have epilepsy or a history of seizures. Do not use if you're a pregnant. Use with medical advice and supervision, if you are nursing. Fennel oil is very powerful and should not be used repeatedly in high doses Do not allow the actual oil into your eyes, nose or ears. Because fennel oil stimulates the secretion of estrogenic hormones, it is not advised for those who currently have or have had breast cancer.

Frankincense Essential Oil:

Frankincense has been valued since ancient times and its essential oil is now known to be a cure for many illnesses and conditions. Frankincense oil has a delicious, woody, deeply spicy aroma that is even better than the scent of frankincense resin.

For Renewal and Anti-Aging: Frankincense oil is so powerful that inhaling it can cause your cells to regenerate and can renew your entire body. It is a renowned beautifier of skin and can slow down the visible signs of aging, such as fine lines, deep lines and wrinkles. Aging skin rapidly begins to lose moisture and becomes dry fragile and cracked. Frankincense oil can combat this by helping skin to regain and retain precious moisture and causing it to look plump, fresh and young again. On the skin of the body, frankincense oil is popular for removing, preventing and reducing the appearance of stretch marks. When skin is scarred, frankincense promotes the regrowth of new skin cells in the damaged area and causes the scar to fade away.

For its Strengthening and Anti-Bleeding Properties: Frankincense oil is a great healer. It has deeply astringent effects that allow it to prevent and slow excessive wound bleeding. It exhibits the ability to quickly heal damage such as cuts wounds and sores. Its anti-bleeding benefits can also help sore and inflamed gums by displaying an astringent effect that heals the affected areas.

For its Anti-Septic Properties: As a strong anti-septic, frankincense oil can remove bacteria and other pollutants from wounds, scratches and cuts, as well as be used as a deep-cleaning agent for surfaces.

For Inflammation Relief: Those suffering with inflammation from autoimmune disorders such as rheumatoid arthritis often report a huge reduction in pain, swelling, stiffness and other signs of inflammation after using frankincense oil.

For Preventing and Healing Colds and Flus: Because frankincense oil is a major expectorant, it helps to break up thick mucus and allows it to be removed from the lungs, throat and nasal airways. Because it is also a disinfectant, breathing in the perfumed air of frankincense oil reduces the germ count in your body and helps you to heal faster and more completely.

For Cancer Prevention: Researchers have found that there are special compounds within frankincense oil that are highly carcinogenic. Not only does frankincense oil help to keep cancer from forming, once it has formed, this oil is unusually adept at causing cancer cells to destroy themselves. In this way, frankincense oil may be one of the most important natural aromatherapy treatments to indulge in, as it could greatly lower cancer risk.

Aromatherapy: Frankincense oil is primarily diffused using a vaporizer or inhaled, in aromatherapy. When used in a steam nebulizer, its scented vapors can offer a calming, sedative effect. Breathing in the essential oil is very effective because doctors believe that frankincense oil acts directly on the brain's limbic system and other areas, providing better cognitive abilities and easing worry and tension. Adding 10 to 15 drops of the oil to bath water or 7 drops into a foot soak, diluting it with a natural base oil such as almond or jojoba oil for a massage oil or simply rubbing it into areas of stiffness and pain can heal aches and inflammation. Applying it in diluted form to problem skin will result in a clearer, softer and more glowing complexion.

Precautions to Remember: Frankincense oil has been in use throughout history and is an incredibly safe and helpful essential oil. However, it is best to avoid it if you are on blood thinning medication because the oil itself may thin the blood. Those who are pregnant or nursing should avoid using frankincense oil in any form because it affects blood flow and spasms of the uterus. If taking frankincense oil internally, make sure to dilute one drop in one glass of water, for protection from irritation. Do not allow children to ingest frankincense oil as it may be too strong for their systems.

Chapter 7

G.

<u>Ginger Oil:</u>

Ginger oil is one of the most beneficial essential oils to have in your cupboard. Distilled from the medicinal ginger root, ginger oil is an amazingly anti-inflammatory and energizing oil.

For Digestive Relief: Because of its warming and balancing powers, ginger oil can be used to relive any digestive problems and return the digestive system to a neutral state. To heal a wide range of digestive troubles from indigestion, gas and nausea to diarrhea and a lost appetite, simply massage a single drop of ginger oil into your stomach area.

For Anti-Inflammatory and Anti-Bacterial Protection: Because ginger oil is made up of 90 percent sesquiterpenes, its anti-inflammatory and healing powers are unrivalled. Sesquiterpenes are also highly antibacterial making ginger oil a great choice to use in a variety of bacterial infections and conditions that cause high fevers. Inhaling a few drops of ginger oil can help you to lower a high body temperature and fight off a respiratory infection. Ginger oil is great for treating flus, coughs, cases of asthma, and bronchitis. Breathing in ginger oil can help to loosen and remove excess mucus from the lungs.

For Food Poisoning: Because ginger oil is highly anti-septic, a few drops can help to treat cases of food poisoning and stomach flu. Its pro-digestive effects also help to ease the nausea and flatulence hat often accompanies these conditions.

For Pain Relief: Ginger oil acts to relieve pain by reducing pain-causing compounds in the body, called prostaglandins. Using ginger oil to massage tender or sore areas will help to alleviate pain and swelling.

For Heart Protection – Studies show that regularly using ginger oil helps to lower the risk of developing blood clots and also lowers levels of bad cholesterol in the body. Ginger oil also has an anti-arteriosclerosis effect on the heart, making it fantastic for all-round heart health.

Aromatherapy: To relieve aches, arthritis, fractures and other pains, add 2 drops of ginger oil into one ounce of base oil and massage the affected areas. To revitalize the body and improve the circulation, use this same blend for a healing all-over massage.

Make a warming winter bath for protection against colds and infections by placing 8 drops of ginger oil into a tub filled with warm water and soak for at least half an hour. As you soak, concentrate on taking deep aromatic breaths. If you don't have time for a full bath, simply place a few drops of the oil on a warm compress and apply to your chest and neck area.

If you are already sick with a cold or suffering from allergies, inhale the steam of the ginger oil by placing a couple of drops on a vaporizer. As you breathe in the vapors, any backed up mucus will begin to flow freely.

Precautions to Remember: When used in the right concentration, ginger oil is one of the safest essential oils of all. Although ginger oil has sometimes been used for morning sickness, all pregnant or nursing women should only use this oil under medical supervision. To dilute ginger oil properly, add it to a suitable carrier oil. The best carrier oils to blend ginger oil with include rose oil, bergamot oil and olive oil.

Ginger oil can cause photosensitivity, so be sure to limit or avoid sun exposure to areas of skin that you've applied the oil to within the last 24 hours. Very young children may be more sensitive than adults so avoid using ginger oil on them. Make sure that you do not overuse ginger oil. Using it every day or in excessive amounts for a prolonged period could result in nausea, skin rashes, mouth sores or other signs of sensitization. If you are taking any prescription medication or have a pre-existing condition, consult with your doctor before using ginger oil.

Grapefruit Oil:

Grapefruit oil is famous for its intensely energizing, protective and weight loss benefits. If you're in need of an essential oil that gives you results you can see, quickly, then this is the choice for you! Grapefruit oil is packed with many of the same properties of whole grapefruits and one of these properties is the ability to aid and support easy weight loss.

Chapter 8:

H.

Hyssop Oil:

Uses of Hyssop Oil

Aromatherapy: Add 5 drops of hyssop oil in ½ a cup of warm water and use this mixture to bathe cuts, wounds, bruises and skin infections. The anti-septic and anti-bacterial effects of hyssop oil will cleanse the area, promote faster healing and prevent sepsis.

Place 3 drops of hyssop oil into an ounce of olive oil and use this blend for a full body massage. This will relieve fatigue as well as all kinds of muscle aches and pains. If you don't have time for a full body massage, simply use the blend for a foot rub and you'll still reap the benefits. You can also apply this same blend to the abdominal area using circular motions and it will effectively relieve stomach cramps and digestive problems.

Add 2 drops of hyssop oil into half an ounce of coconut oil and rub this into the feet for a quick fever reducing remedy that works quickly.

Placing 2 drops of hyssop oil in a cup of water and using this mixture on the skin can help rashes, mosquito and insect bites and even boils to heal.

When this hyssop mix is used on scars, it can speed up scar fading and help to rejuvenate the skin. To speed up the scar facing process even more, add a drop of hyssop oil to an unscented, natural-based lotion and apply to the area.

Add 2 drops of hyssop oil to a nebulizer and deeply inhale the steam, for a revitalizing and healing treatment that will remove excess mucus and cleanse the respiratory tract.

Precautions to Remember: It's important to keep in mind that while hyssop oil has many benefits, it is a very potent substance. Because hyssop can contain high levels of pinocamphone, it can be toxic to the body if used in large amounts. For this reason, it is vital to always use hyssop oil in moderation and to seek the opinion of and professional aromatherapist or doctor.

Hyssop oil's pinocamphone content could also cause epilepsy and should not be used by epileptics. Hyssop oil may be highly toxic for children and could result in fever, epilepsy or skin damage, so it should only be used by adults. Pregnant and nursing women should avoid taking or using hyssop oil in any form unless advised otherwise by their physician. Because hyssop oil can raise blood pressure, those with hypertension should avoid using hyssop oil.

Always dilute hyssop oil in a carrier oil before applying topically, to avoid skin irritation and sensitivity. Almond and coconut oil are the best choices to dilute hyssop oil with.

Chapter 9

I.

Idaho Blue Spruce Oil:

From weight issues to aches, the refreshing and soothing essential oil of Idaho blue spruce can be used as a fast acting remedy for many different health problems.

For Weight Loss: If you're trying to lose weight and need an extra boost beyond diet and exercise, adding Idaho blue spruce oil to your fitness plan can help. In aromatherapy, this oil is widely used to shed unwanted weight in a targeted way. Idaho blue spruce oil is able to rapidly lower the amount of brown fat within your body. This is important because brown fat is the type of fat that is often referred to as internal. It is a visceral fat that doesn't simply sit on your body's surface but actually wraps itself around your most delicate organs, dislocating them and causing inflammation and permanent damage.

Idaho blue spruce oil works against brown fat because it is packed with citral a natural, brown fat–busting substance that quickly cuts down on this dangerous type of adipose tissue. The benefits of Idaho blue spruce oil can be accessed in both topical massages and internal consumption.

For Pain Relief: Idaho blue spruce oil is a powerful anti-inflammatory substance. It exhibits a highly analgesic, pain-killing effect. Used in moderate doses, it has shown the ability to reduce and even completely relieve everything from toothaches to deep nerve pain.

For Muscular Pain Soothing Properties: Using Idaho blue spruce oil in a bath or diluted as a massage oil can help to loosen, worn out or tight muscles as well as relieve built up nervous tension. If you suffer from chronic migraines or TMJ jaw and facial pain, using this oil for a deep tissue rub can smooth out constricted joints. It quickly eases cramped muscles and can be a great way to manage and get rid of chronic pain. For a quick dose of this pain relief, simply take a whiff of the oil, from the bottle during your day, for immediate relief from fatigue and soreness. When doing so, make sure that you keep the bottle at least 5 inches away when inhale the scent, to avoid overpowering your nose. Because Idaho blue spruce oil is excellent at easing deep tissue pain, it is a wonderfully healing treatment option for fibromyalgia sufferers who do not exhibit allergic reactions to strong scents.

For Testosterone Levels: Many men find that with age their testosterone levels dip quickly. This is a part of andropause but while natural, it can cause fatigue, stress, weight gain, muscle loss, aging skin and other health problems. However, simply adding 3 drops of Idaho blue spruce oil in a glass of water, to your daily regimen can help to increase testosterone levels by as much as 30% over a couple of months!

Aromatherapy: To balance the body and help to fight low testosterone levels, place 5 drops of Idaho blue spruce oil on the soles of the feet and massage the oil in well. Do this up to 2 times a week to see a real difference. To ease muscle tension and reduce stress levels, add 2 drops of Idaho blue spruce oil and 2 drops of Idaho balsam fir oil into a warm foot bath and soak for at least 15 minutes. When you need to get rid of a headache or backache quickly, simply place 1 drop of Idaho blue spruce oil into the palm of your hand. Rub both hands together to intensify the scent and breathe in deeply. This refreshing and energizing essential oil can relax you and naturally banish all forms of pain.

Precautions to Remember: Idaho blue spruce oil could cause sensitization or irritation if used too frequently, so try to space out usage. Never use the oil undiluted, instead blend it with a carrier oil or pure water for best effects. It is not advised for young children or pregnant and nursing women to use Idaho blue spruce essential oil.

While this oil is generally considered safe for consumption, make sure to consult with your doctor before doing so, in order to avoid any allergic reactions. This oil may be toxic to cats, so please keep it away from pets.

Chapter 10

J.

Jasmine Essential Oil:

Jasmine oil is one of the most highly valued essential oils of all. It is often called jasmine absolute, due to its special extraction methods and offers a wonderfully sweet and floral fragrance as well as many important healing applications.

For Abdominal Cramps: Jasmine oil can relax and soothe tene or cramping muscle s in the stomach area. Simply apply 2 drops of the oil to your abdominal skin and massage in a gentle circular motion, for deep pain relief.

For Hair Health: To add a nourishing natural sheen to dry or damaged hair, use jasmine essential oil in the place of other synthetic products. Add 2 drops of the oil to your palms and rub together vigorously before applying the warmed oil from root to tip. Doing this several times a week will result in healthier more manageable and vibrant hair.

For an extra luxurious treat, try adding 3 drops of jasmine oil to your usual conditioner. Massage this mixture into the scalp and hair and allow it to absorb for 10 minutes before rinsing out.

For Dry Skin: Jasmine oil is particularly good for revitalizing fry, cracked, wrinkled and aging skin. To harness the youth renewing properties of this oil, place 2 drops of it on any dry, rough or wrinkled areas and pat well into the skin to allow proper absorption. Follow this with your usual nightly moisturizer. As I've mentioned before, I don't recommend using essential oils on the skin during the day because any contact with sunlight could lead to irritation or damage, so please make sure to enjoy this skin treatment in the evenings only for best results.

For Depression or Anxiousness: The jasmine flower is known to produce a particularly calming and cheerful scent. According to research, jasmine oil has actually been linked to the release of serotonin within the brain, allowing this feel-good hormone to positively impact the mental state of those who inhale the scent.

For Wound Cleansing: Jasmine oil is also an amazingly effective disinfectant and anti-septic oil. It contains potent germ, bacteria virus and fungus killing substances such as benzaldehyde, benzyl benzoate and benzoic acid. Applying 4 drops of it to a half-cup of warm water and rinsing any open wounds or cuts with this mixture will prevent infection, sepsis and even speed up healing. You can also access the anti-cold, anti-flu and respiratory infection-fighting action of this oil by simply inhaling its fragrance.

For Scars and Stretchmarks: Jasmine oil can quickly heal damaged skin and can even quickly erase all evidence of scars and stretchmarks. Although treating newer scars and stretchmarks works best, this oil is powerful enough to alleviate the appearance of even very old scars and marks. If you have stubborn marks and discolorations that seem to resist al conventional fade creams, try dabbing 1 drop of jasmine oil on them and massaging the area gently. Do this up to 3 times a week and you will notice that the marks will start to fade away on their own. As an added plus, jasmine oil's all natural components will do the job without any harsh chemicals to irritate the delicate scar tissue!

Aromatherapy: Add 2 drops of jasmine oil to a diffuser and allow the scent to circulate freely. Breathe the scent in deeply for both relaxation and a boost to your immune system. Place 3 drops of jasmine oil in an ounce of coconut oil and massage the skin thoroughly for a stress-relieving treatment that will leave your mind calm and make your skin supple, glowing and firm.

Precautions to Remember: Because it is an emmenagogue, jasmine oil can overstimulate the uterus and should therefore be avoided by pregnant women. When using this oil in a diffuser or nebulizer, be careful to limit the amount you apply, because it has almost sedative-like qualities and can cause sleepiness, fatigue and confusion. Use no more than 3 drops for steam or vapor inhalation purposes.

Juniper Oil:

Juniper oil is a deliciously fresh and vibrant oil that can be used in so many great ways! It has been prized for its health promoting compounds since ancient and modern research shows that it richly deserves this reputation.

For its Astringent Properties: Juniper oil possesses strong astringent qualities that help it do so much, from healing tooth and gum pain, to preventing hair loss and even halting diarrhea. If you ever find yourself suffering from cramps and having to run to the bathroom constantly, simply inhaling one whiff of juniper oil can provide you with instant relief!

For its Deeply Detoxifying Nature: This oil is known to be a "depurative"or blood cleansing agent. It quickly removes all traces of toxins from the blood, purifying out everything from heavy metals to chemicals and uric acid, while supporting the kidney's elimination process. It also helps the body to perspire properly, allowing for maximum detoxification. Through these properties, juniper oil provides a deep and complete cleansing and detoxing effect that will balance your body and can even promote proper weight loss. As a result, using juniper oil while going on a cleanse, juice fast or diet can make your efforts more successful.

For its Carminative Properties: Juniper oil is also a useful digestive aid, helping to push gas downward and out of the body, instead of allowing it to remain trapped in the chest area. As a carminative agent this oil also promotes digestive stability and discourages any extra gas from forming. These traits make it a helpful supplementary treatment for anyone who regularly suffers from bloating and flatulence.

For its Tonic Effects: Only the most active, health-giving substances are considered to be tonics and juniper oil completely fits the bill.as an effective cleanser, sudorific, digestive and stimulant, this oil can be used to gain and maintain overall health and fitness. When inhaled, it cleanses and strengthens the respiratory tract and when used topically, it protects and stabilizes the entire bod. To put it simply you can't really go wrong when using juniper oil for healing.

Aromatherapy: For an air purifying and disinfectant effect, add 4 drops of juniper oil to a diffuser. For a quick body boosting treatment that will truly draw out deep-seated toxins and impurities from the blood and organs through the skin, you can mix 5 drops of juniper oil into one ounce of jojoba oil and use this blend while dry brushing the entire body. Use firm, sweeping strokes to work the juniper in and to help release all pollutants.

To immediately quell nausea, diarrhea or pain, place 1 drop of juniper oil on clean cotton ball and take a bracing sniff!

Precautions to Remember: Juniper oil is not only regarded as one of the most useful essential oils but also one of the very safest. In order to avoid any potential complications, be sure to use it after diluting in water or oil and always in low doses. Those with kidney problems or those who are pregnant should not use juniper oil.

Chapter 11
L.

Lavender Oil:

The root of the name lavender actually means "to wash" so it's really no surprise that lavender essential oil is one of the best natural cleansers around. This oil has a lovely, mildly spiced, floral scent that has been a favorite in aromatherapy and healing treatments for many years.

For Cleansing: True to its name, the potent cleansing powers of lavender oil make it excellent for treating the bacteria that is responsible for causing acne and also for cleansing the scalp and hair thoroughly. In the case of acne, this painful and distressing skin condition is the result of an excess of sebum production as well as an overgrowth of harmful bacteria feeding off of the excessive sebum. When applied on acne prone skin, lavender oil sinks deep into the dermis to combat and kill off the dangerous bacteria and reduce inflammation, leaving the skin clear and clean. Lavender oil also works on the scalp by removing lice eggs, full grown lice and nits. It purifies the scalp of all pathogens and sets the stage for the growth of thick, healthy hair.

For Chronic Pain: Many people who experience chronic pain believe that they are doomed to continue taking powerful prescription pain killers for many years, but lavender oil can be a great, inexpensive and healthy alternative. Whether you suffer from arthritis, autoimmune-led joint and muscle pain or simply a bad back, you can get genuine relief by making a bottle of lavender oil your go to pain killer. According to research, when lavender oil was added to the air in hospital rooms where postoperative patients were resting, they reported experiencing less pain and recovered from their surgeries faster than usual

To get these results for yourself, all you need to do is periodically smell the scent wafting from your bottle of pure lavender oil.

For Good Blood Flow: If your blood is circulating sluggishly, many tests suggest that the scent of lavender oilcan help. It appears to have a markedly positive effect on blood flow around the body and can even reduce high blood pressure levels in hypertension patients. Lavender oil's ability to improve coronary circulation translates into tons of benefits for the entire body. Good blood flow allows organs to receive the right amount of oxygen, gives the brain's functions a helping hand and heals the heart, preventing the development of serious cardiac diseases.

For Great Sleep: Lavender has always traditionally been used to treat sleeping disorders and because lavender oil is a more concentrated form of the plant, its sleep improving qualities are even stronger. Due to its soft, calming fragrance, it affects the autonomic nervous system and balances out the heart rate. In fact, repeated studies have shown that when insomniacs replace their usual sleep medication with the scent of lavender, they enjoy deeper, less interrupted sleep. Using lavender oil not only boosts the quality of sleep, it also increases the long term regularity of sleep, making it the perfect way to get great, restful sleep naturally.

For Brain Benefits: Lavender oil's relaxing effects aren't limited to fixing sleep problems either. It can help just as much in the waking hours. According to several studies, students who breathed in the scent of lavender oil before taking an exam all showed less anxiety, nervousness and stress and also exhibited improved brain functioning, while taking the exam.

For its Insect Repellant Powers: This oil is also a super insect repellant. The scent of lavender oil is enough to ward off moths, bugs and mosquitoes, making it a safe alternative to conventional bug sprays. In fact, lavender oil works so well that many bug sprays contain large amounts of it in their formula.

Aromatherapy: To relieve tension and improve sleep, add 3 to 5 drops of lavender oil to a warm compress and apply to the forehead. Do this at least 15 minutes before trying to sleep and you'll find yourself drifting off easily. To access the brain and blood flow-boosting benefits of this oil, simply add 3 drops of it to a diffuser and breathe in the scent. To keep mosquitoes away as you sleep, simply dab a few drops of the oil onto your pillows and bedsheets.

Precautions to Remember: Lavender essential oil should NEVER be ingested internally. Consuming lavender oil orally can result in nausea, vomiting, breathing problems, blurred vision and diarrhea. As amazing as this awesome oil is, it is very important to only use it topically or as an aromatherapy scent, via a diffuser or nebulizer.

Lavender oil must never be used by people with diabetes or those who are pregnant or nursing. Always test your tolerance of lavender oil by doing a patch test beforehand and avoid overusing the oil or using it in larger amounts, as this could increase intolerance and cause a reaction.

Chapter 12

M.

Marjoram Oil: Marjoram oil is filled with important components including alpha terpinene, linalool, sabinene and many other active substances that have been identified as good for overall health. Marjoram oil is widely used in the Mediterranean region to treat various ailments and conditions

For Protection against Viruses and Infections: Marjoram oil's active substances are all highly anti-viral and anti-bacterial. Using this oil can offer real protection from a variety of influenza virus strains, measles, a range of pox types and can even fight off the common cold. As an intense bacteria killer, marjoram oil can aid in preventing and treating many different types of bacterial infections, including food poisoning and skin conditions. It can also be used to quickly and thoroughly cleanse the infectious air of sickrooms.

For Brain Rejuvenation: Marjoram oil is well-known as a cephalic substance, meaning that it provides protective and rejuvenating effects to the brain. While the brain naturally loses its vitality as part of the aging process, using marjoram essential oil can help to slow and even keep many of these cognitive losses at bay. It appears to increase the quantity of blood flow to the brain, therefore reducing the risk of damage from age-related cerebral diseases like Alzheimer's and Parkinson's and keeping the brain young and active into the future.

For Weight Loss and Detox: This oil increases the body's ability to perspire and urinate, allowing your system to fully purge out unnecessary items like built up sodium salts and toxins. As urination increases, marjoram oil helps you to expel excess fat. It also promotes the loss of bloated water weight, giving you a light feeling. Marjoram oil also acts as a febrifuge, working to cool off any hidden inflammatory fevers within the body through its detoxifying effects.

For Digestive Health: The marjoram plant was always used as a digestive throughout the centuries and we now know that its digestive powers are entirely in its essential oils. Using marjoram oil helps you to totally rebalance your digestive system, ensuring the right amount of vital digestive substances such as bile, acids and gastric juices are all released at the right times and in the right amounts . Marjoram oil is also able to cause the intestines to move and contract in a way that is good for digestion. As it stimulates these movements, food is then able to pass through the intestines in a timely manner. This oil also has a naturally laxative effect, meaning that with proper usage, bowel movements become regular and the whole digestive system stays healthy.

For Speedy Muscle Repair: If you've ever pulled a muscle, you know just how excruciating and hard to heal that issue is. But while over the counter rubs don't always work fast or well enough, simply adding a couple of drops of marjoram oil to your regular lotion and giving yourself a gentle rub will have you feeling as good as new in no time.

For Anti-Aging: Premature aging can be brought on by everything from smoking to dehydration and lack of sleep but when it comes to erasing the signs of aging from the skin, few oils work as well as marjoram. That's because marjoram oil is extremely high in antioxidants. When applied to the skin in a diluted solution of 2 drops marjoram oil to an ounce of jojoba or coconut oil, this oil's antioxidants literally go scavenging for any free radicals, preventing damage to the complexion and even turning back the clock on preexisting damage.

For Cardiac Protection: As a well-known hypotensive, marjoram oil can provide a safe and gentle healing option for high blood pressure levels. Along with following any professional medical advice provided by your doctor, adding 2-3 drops of this wonderful oil to a carrier oil like olive oil and indulging in a full body massage using this blend several times a week can help drop blood pressure and cut the risk of heart attacks, strokes and bleeding of the brain.

For Snoring: Another surprising but very useful application of marjoram oil is in snoring prevention. If you or a loved one can't seem to get through the night without snoring, gasping for breath or experiencing sleep apnea, try marjoram oil for its ability to relax the respiratory system and prevent these and other nighttime breathing disturbances.

Aromatherapy: To get rid of headaches, nervous tension and muscle aches, use 2 drops of marjoram in 1 ounce of olive oil. You can add the blend to each temple and rub gently or even try a shoulder and neck massage. For all over relief, add 3 drops instead of 2 and use the blend in a full body massage. You can also use this recipe in a cool or warm compress for lumbago and other types of back pain. If you're suffering from digestive issues such as indigestion, excessive gas or constipation, apply 3 drops of marjoram to a carrier oil and rub gently on the back. For general pain relief and cardiac health, add 8-9 drops of marjoram oil to a running bath and soak for half an hour. To get rid of snoring, try adding a single drop of marjoram oil to your pillow. If this doesn't provide immediate results, you can also place a drop of diluted marjoram oil on the upper lip or even a mustache, to allow all night inhalation. Another great use for marjoram oil is as an anti-nausea and anti-spasmodic application for car or seasickness. Simply put 2 drops of pure marjoram oil on a clean handkerchief and smell periodically.

Precautions to Remember: Avoid using marjoram oil if pregnant or nursing. Do not use in children or those who are clinically depressed as the oil's strongly sedative effect may prove negative in such cases. Avoid using marjoram oil in high doses or frequently, as this could cause confusion and sleepiness. Be careful when operating heavy machinery or driving, after marjoram oil use.

Chapter 13

N.

Nutmeg Oil:

Nutmeg oil is steam distilled from nutmeg, a fruit that is native to the Moluccas or Spice Islands. This amazingly fragrant and enticing essential oil has captured the imagination and desires of many throughout the centuries and for very good reasons: With benefits that range from banishing bad breath to promoting detoxification, nutmeg oil should be at the top of your list for a spicy scented natural treatment that can heal, balance and renew.

For its Phytochemical Content: Nutmeg oil is filled with important phytochemicals such as tannins, flavonoids, glycosides, phenolics, alkaloids and steroids. These ingredients are so active and powerful that they have been found to exert highly anti-microbial effects against many different types of dangerous pathogens. So if you want to ward off E.coli and other deadly strains of infectious pathogens, keeping nutmeg oil around is a definite bonus.

For its Reportedly Anti-Cancer Effects: According to several studies carried out on animals, nutmeg oil could be one of nature's overlooked anti-carcinogenic treatments. This oil contains many essential compounds that seem to block the actions of hazardous carcinogen-promoting enzymes.

For its Ability to Treat Bad Breath: Halitosis, or bad breath, is a very uncomfortable condition that requires urgent and effective treatment. Cue nutmeg oil! Nutmeg oil works against bad breath using a two pronged approach. It is highly scented, anti-bacterial and can remove any fungal remnants in the mouth while masking any unpleasant odors. At the same time, it works on a deeper level as well, by allowing its scent to enter the gut and eliminate the toxins and pathogens that may be the secret underlying cause of the bad breath in the first place. By gargling with a diluted nutmeg oil solution, you can achieve instantly fresher breath while also allowing the substance to root out the real cause of the problem at the same time.

For a Powerfully Detoxifying Treatment: Use this oil when you need to give your regular detox or juice cleanse a serious boost. Nutmeg oil works efficiently to pull up, draw out and eliminate built up toxins from all organs and the liver and kidneys, in particular. Within the kidneys, it acts to cure infections and inflammatory conditions. It also has the ability to aid in dissolving harmful waste byproducts such as uric acid and promotes the full removal of these substances, leaving the body cleansed and ready for better health.

For a Soothing Massage: Try substituting your usual massage oil for nutmeg essential oil blended into a carrier oil. Doing so will help to smooth out any cricks, constricted muscles and stiff joints. It works very well as an after-work out oil treatment and women can also use it to deal with the deep muscular pain and inflammation that occurs during menstruation. When using this oil, not only are you soothing your body but you are also adding natural anti-bacterial and anti-pathogenic protection to your skin, so go ahead and concentrate on areas such as spaces between the toes and skin folds, where warm, covered conditions could breed unwanted germs.

Aromatherapy: To eliminate bad breath, place 1-2 drops of nutmeg in comfortably warm water and gargle thoroughly with this mix. Doing this 2-3 times a week will help to get rid of halitosis and the bacteria that cause it. To heal digestive problems, speed up detoxification of the kidneys and soothe a worn out body, add 7 drops of nutmeg oil to a warm bath and enjoy a long soak. You can also gain improved focus, mental clarity and improved breathing by adding 4 drops of nutmeg oil to a nebulizer and breathing the resulting steam in deeply.

Precautions to Remember: It is critical to keep in mind that nutmeg oil is only for topical use and should not be consumed orally.

Because this oil is highly concentrated and very potent, you should never use it in undiluted form. Instead, dilute it with good carrier oils such as coconut oil, olive oil, jojoba oil or almond oil. You may have heard about nutmeg's hallucinogenic properties. Because nutmeg contains myristicin, it can lead in some cases, to hallucinations and other unpleasant side effects. However, nutmeg essential oil typically contains about 4% myristicin and is generally considered safe when applied topically, inhaled in very low doses and not used too frequently in a limited time span. Those with epilepsy should not use nutmeg oil as it is a strong stimulant. Pregnant and nursing women as well as children should not use nutmeg oil in any form.

Ingesting nutmeg oil can lead to dangerous side effects so be sure to use this oil only as advised. When nutmeg oil is used in inhalations, make sure that you use a very moderate amount as too much can also lead to delirium, excessive sleep, convulsions and visual problems. If you have any questions or concerns, it's always best to seek out professional medical advice when using this powerful oil.

Chapter 14
O.

Orange Essential Oil:

Orange oil is a superstar in the aromatherapy world because it has so many different beneficial properties. It is an anti-spasmodic, anti-inflammatory, anti-septic, carminative, tonic, diuretic and sedative oil, just to name a few of its uses. Let's look at some of the best reasons to use this intense essential oil:

For its Sedative and Relaxing Qualities: Nothing takes the edge off a stressful day or relieves a backlog of tension and anxiety like orange oil. As a pulse rate-decreasing agent, this pure and natural substance can do the work of an anti-depressant or anti-anxiety medication while helping you to avoid the many physical risks of long term prescription medication use. Orange oil works by calming systemic inflammation within the body and mind, to relieve pent-up stress.

For its Antiseptic Powers: Using orange oil in a diluted water bath to wash wounds, cuts and insect bites is an effective way of ensuring the area stays safe from bacterial infection. Because the compounds in this oil are great at fighting off dangerous microbes and fungi, orange oil is an ideal choice for cleansing wounds and preventing sepsis, tetanus and fungal infections.

For its Diuretic Abilities: This oil will have you heading to the bathroom frequently, but trust me, this is one of its best properties. Because orange oil is highly diuretic, it helps your body to release much of its toxicity through urination. If you suffer from sallow skin and a bitter taste in the mouth, you may have a problem with excessive bile production.

Inhaling the scent of this oil for can help to stimulate the desire for urination and therefore, eliminate the backlog of bile. Allergy sufferers can access another great benefit of orange oil's diuretic effect, because frequent urination can also help to clear inflammation and stored allergens in the system.

For its Anti-Dementia Benefits: Research has shown that using orange essential oil in aromatherapy treatments like massages and diffusions can positively impact the cognitive abilities of those who suffer from various types of dementia, including Alzheimer's Disease.

Aromatherapy: A fantastic essential oil for newcomers to the world of aromatherapy, orange oil allows for many beneficial uses and is both inexpensive and generally quite safe, so beginners can enjoy trying out lots of blends and treatments. For healthy, bacteria-free skin, add 1-2 drops of orange oil to a moistened cotton ball and sweep gently over the skin. Add 2-3 drops of the oil to a diffuser and enjoy the anti-depressant and stress lifting properties of the scent. For anti-inflammatory and febrifuge benefits, add 3-4 drops to a cool compress and apply to the forehead. To relieve the respiratory tract during a cold or flu, blend 2-3 drops of the oil into olive or almond oil and rub gently over the chest and upper back area. To ease fluid retention and bloating, add 8-9 drops to a warm bath and soak.

Precautions to Remember: Do not expose orange oil treated skin to sunlight within 24 hours of treatment, as this may result in photosensitivity and blemishes. As with all essential oils, pregnant and nursing women should avoid this oil unless advised otherwise by their doctors. Although quite safe, this and other essential oils are not recommended for young children without medical supervision. Although orange oil is often consumed in packaged foods and beverages, overconsumption could lead to indigestion and stomach upset.

Oregano Oil:

Oregano oil is a disinfectant, anti-parasitic, anti-fungal and anti-bacterial oil. It has been used since ancient times in Greece, for its cleaning and purifying abilities. Historically, oregano oil was employed to cleanse wounds and treat food poisoning and bacterial infections and today, those same buses still apply. Oregano oil is unique in that, it works fantastically in a variety of ways, whether applied topically, inhaled or ingested in very low doses with honey or properly diluted in water.

For its Anti-Parasitic Properties: The human body is very vulnerable to attacks by a variety of parasitic organisms, ranging from tape and roundworms to lice, bedbugs and fleas. A parasitic infestation is a true health nightmare and requires urgent action but unfortunately, many of the anti- parasitic medicaments on the market today are just as harsh to human health as they are to the parasites they are meant to remove. In the case of an infestation, why not try oregano oil? Known since ancient times for its cleansing powers, this oil is also a prolific parasite killer!

Ingesting a small amount of oregano oil, diluted in a suitable carrier such as water, honey, or another non-dairy substance, can help to destroy worms and internal bacteria. When you apply this oil to the skin and scalp, it is equally good at repelling lice, mites and fleas. And because this oil is natural, you can use it without the fear of ingesting dangerous chemicals!

For its Autoimmune Regulation: Oregano oil can rebalance and calm the immune functions of the body, allowing those who suffer from autoimmune diseases to gain relief from the constant pain of their conditions. Because this oil regulates the behavior of white blood cells, it is good for both soothing an overactive immune system and rousing a weakened or damaged one.

For its Fantastic Phenols: This oil is packed with plenty of phenols, making it one of the best free radical fighters out there. While protecting against any new free radical damage to your body and skin, it also fends off any new attack and can help in preventing several conditions. These include premature aging, vision damage, hearing problems, loss of muscle mass and long term nerve damage. Because of its ability to keep all of these and other conditions at bay, oregano oil has become known as the preferred essential oil to use in the fight against aging. Even more importantly, its high phenol content is also a potent anti-carcinogenic, showing promise in research that this oil can be used to prevent many different types of cancer, especially those of the skin.

Aromatherapy: Add 5 drops of oregano oil to 2 teaspoons of almond oil and blend well. Use this as a powerful massage oil that can be applied all over the body for anti-septic, anti-bacterial and antioxidant benefits. Add 1-2 drops of oregano oil to a glass of water and drink this mixture for relief from viral and bacterial respiratory infections. This drink also makes a great sore throat soother, as well. Because oregano oil is highly concentrated and strong, don't add it directly to broken, infected skin. Instead, mix 3 drops of the oil into 1 teaspoon of olive oil and apply tis to areas that require oregano oil's antiseptic cleansing. You can also diffuse 3 drops of oregano oil and enjoy the calming, fresh and woody fragrance, for relaxation.

Precautions to Remember: Because oregano oil is a known emmenagogue, pregnant women should avoid using oregano oil in any form, to prevent dangerous uterine stimulation, hormone stimulation and other risks.

Using the oil topically in high doses could result in irritation and allergy. While oregano oil is excellent for health when consumed in low doses, it is important to avoid taking high doses of this potent oil. Consult with a doctor before using this oil on young children and always dilute this oil with a good carrier oil or clean water, before topical application.

Chapter 15

P.

Patchouli Oil:

An extremely versatile oil, patchouli is beloved for its sedative, anti-depressant, anti-microbial and health-promoting effects. You can use patchouli oil in a number of truly incredible ways!

For its Insect Repellant Properties: Patchouli oil is a well-known insecticide and bug repellant. Because it is an all-natural substance, using it in place of store-bought repellants can provide relief from insects in a safe, healthy way.

For its Cytophylactic Properties: Did you know that this essential stands head and shoulders above all the rest, because of its renewing abilities? Patchouli oil is a proven regenerator of the body through its ability to cause the creation and growth of brand new cells! Patchouli oil is also a red blood cell promoter, thereby increasing the energy levels and overall vitality of those who use it. Once it helps to create new cells, this oil doesn't stop there. In fact, it enhances circulation and ensures that all cells and organs receive an adequate supply of oxygen, through oxygenation of the entire body. With these mechanisms, this oil is also an excellent metabolism booster and contributes to the appearance of a firm, young and smooth complexion.

For its Ability to Fight Fevers: Because inflammation is often at the root of so many modern health problems these days, the ability to calm and soothe inflammation and quench systemic fevers makes patchouli oil a prized and essential treatment.

Whether it is used to cool an internal fever arising from chronic inflammation, such as is commonly found in autoimmune conditions or it is applied topically to cool the fires of dermatological inflammation, patchouli oil simply cannot be matched in its ability to douse the body's inflammatory flames. Try it in a soothing cool compress for skin conditions or in a relaxing soak, to treat autoimmune inflammation.

For Deodorizing: Patchouli oil possesses a strong, musky and spicy fragrance that can effectively remove body odor or environmental odors. When applied topically in a massage, this scent appears to use its antiseptic properties to strip away any odors and replaces them with patchouli's own distinctive and exotic aroma. When you diffuse patchouli oil in a room, it gets rid of any stale or unpleasant smells and also provides an anti-septic living atmosphere.

For its Mood Lifting Qualities: Patchouli oil has always been regarded as an anti-depressant and natural mood lifter but now research backs this folklore up. Studies show that inhaling the aroma of patchouli stimulates the brain to produce and release more of the feel-good hormones serotonin and dopamine, resulting in a more stable, content and cheerful outlook in those who use it.

Aromatherapy: Burn a couple of drops of patchouli oil in a room or closet to keep bugs, mites, mosquitoes and moths away. Make sure to air the rooms thoroughly afterwards, so that everything you own doesn't end up smelling of pure patchouli and be careful with dosage, for the same reason! Make mixture of 9-10 drops of patchouli and ½ cup of warm water and sprinkle this mix on the perimeters of bug infested areas or on actual bug colonies themselves, for a simple and inexpensive insecticide. You can also further dilute this mixture and use it wash sheets, in order to keep bedbugs and fleas at bay. To treat eczema and other skin inflammation conditions, add 7-8 drops of patchouli oil to a warm, not hot, bath and soak for half an hour. Do this 2 times a week, for intensive healing. Massage 4 drops of patchouli mixed into an ounce of coconut oil into your skin, for a purifying and anti-aging treatment.

Precautions to Remember: Patchouli oil is not considered safe for use by pregnant women. It may also cause strong allergic reactions in children, so proceed with caution. The scent of patchouli oil, though pleasant to many, may be too strong for some. Always test your own reaction before applying the oil and remember, when diffusing or using in any way, this oil has a very persistent fragrance that doesn't fade as quickly as those of other oils. Be careful when using it around furnishings and clothing, as the smell may last for quite a while.

Patchouli is quite safe when used in topical or inhaled preparations. This oil doesn't need to be diluted as much as others, but dilution is always best. Try mixing it with lavender or rose oil in a coconut or olive carrier oil for a great blend. Keep patchouli oil far away from your eyes, nose and ears. When used for consumption, patchouli oil can be a true healer. However, it is important to do so only with the advice of a medical professional! This oil should not be consumed by those with digestive issues. Overusing patchouli oil or using it in large amounts can trigger too much stimulation and could result in appetite loss and fatigue. I don't recommend this oil for anyone who is in the first stages of recovering from any illness, as it could contribute to nausea and malaise.

Peppermint Oil:

With its long history of use and sweetly refreshing and enlivening fragrance, peppermint oil has earned its place on the list of top essential oils. While this oil is loved by all aromatherapy buffs, even conventional health practitioners acknowledge its powerfully healing qualities and prescribe it in cases when other medical treatments aren't working. Let's take a look at some of the surprising ways that a few drops of peppermint oil can heal, refresh and revitalize you!

For A Major Dose of Vitamins and Nutrients: While everyone loves this delectably scented oil, few realize that not only does peppermint oil smell good, it also does a body good! It is filled with an awe inspiring amount of nutrients and minerals, such as magnesium, manganese, folate, iron, calcium, copper and potassium. And if that's not enough to make it the queen of oils, take into account its high levels of vitamin C, vitamin A and skin-nourishing omega-3 fatty acids. While most substances require you to consume them internally to provide any lasting nutrient benefits, peppermint oil is different. Simply applying this oil topically a few times a week is enough to garner all of the fantastic anti-aging effects that these oxidation-fighting vitamins and minerals offer.

For Healing of the Digestive System: While numerous essential oils are considered to be good for digestion, none can claim the same level of digestive healing that peppermint oil provides. Since ancient times, people have been turning to this wonderful substance to battle bloating, nausea, heartburn and even the most severe symptoms of irritable bowel syndrome. Nowadays, peppermint oil has been shown to be an instant reliever of motion sickness, a restorer of lost appetites and an excellent carminative substance. It works by releasing tension in the smooth muscles found in the gastrointestinal tract. Peppermint oil is so effective at healing indigestion, bowel spasms, and bowel movement irregularity through this relaxing mechanism that it is often a major ingredient in many of the popular "over-the-counter" medicines available commercially. One easy way to use this oil to soothe chronic heartburn is to add 1 drop of it to 1 drop of caraway oil. These oils can be gently massaged over the chest and upper stomach and exert a calming, balancing effect on troubled stomachs.

For Great Oral Health: Need to add a natural boost to your dental care routine? Look no further than peppermint oil. It possesses strongly anti-septic, anti-microbial and pain-killing compounds that make it an ideal way to give your teeth a little extra looking after. Whether you want to prevent gum disease, fight off a nasty tooth infection or reduce the pain of a procedure at the dentist's office, just inhaling this fragrant oil can help you to achieve all of those aims. Additionally, placing 2-3 drops of the oil into a ½ cup of warm water and swishing this mix thoroughly around the mouth will tighten swollen gums, remove hard-to-reach bacteria and freshen up the breath remarkably. No wonder peppermint oil is a staple ingredient in toothpastes and mouthwashes.

Aromatherapy: To get rid of a severe headache, dilute 3-4 drops of peppermint oil to carrier oil and apply gently to the forehead, temples and jaw line. Doctors often prescribe peppermint oil as a remedy for migraines, when pain killers aren't effective. If you often experience migraines, diffuse the oil and inhale deeply. Its scent and anti-inflammatory nature often work quickly to banish both the headaches and the nausea that they tend to cause within 20 minutes. Apply a diluted blend of peppermint oil and jojoba or olive oil to any hot, swollen or inflamed areas. This oil's ability to impart a cooling sensation can help to bring down fevers and tenderness and many who suffer from sore points throughout the body have benefitted from its anti-heat and anti-pain effects. This cooling quality, when coupled with its anti-septic nature, provides a perfect treatment for the burning and itchiness of dandruff and other scalp conditions. Simply put 2-3 drops of peppermint oil in half a cup of water and use this as a cleansing and purifying rinse. You can also dip a comb in this solution and run it through the hair, for a quick but effective treatment.

Precautions to Remember: Peppermint oil is widely used but some precautions do apply. As with all oils, do a small patch test to check for any allergic reactions before using. Avoid using the oil undiluted and avoid use in pregnant and nursing women. Do not use internally on children and for adults, always consult with a doctor before oral consumption. Using peppermint topically and in low doses is considered to be the safest and most beneficial method of treatment.

Chapter 16

R.

Rose Oil:

 Rose essential oil is steam distilled from the most highly scented and oil-filled roses in the world. This luxuriously aromatic oil has literally hundreds of different active constituents, making it not only beautifully fragrant but also very healthy. Rose oil provides many healing opportunities and can be used in numerous safe and gentle yet powerful blends.

For its Febrifuge Effects: Rose oil is fever fighter. It works on a cellular level to calm the raging flames of inflammation and allows the body and mind to gain much needed relief. Because inflammation is the foundation of modern illness, rose oil can be used to prevent and address such issues as diabetes, autoimmune disorders, depression and dementia. While smelling pure rose oil works well to soothe cerebral inflammation, soaking in a bath of 7-8 drops of rose oil in room temperature water can ensure that the anti-inflammatory and febrifuge effects are able to reach all parts of the body.

For its Antiviral Protection: Viruses are highly contagious and difficult to treat so the best possible line of defense is prevention. Rose oil provides this prevention by effectively guarding the mucus membranes from airborne viruses such as the flu. This preventative effect has been studied and is considered an important finding because unlike so many medications, rose oil's natural antiviral properties are able to withstand the many mutations that viruses undergo and continue to offer comprehensive protection, flu season after flu season.

For its Skin Rejuvenating Effects: Historically, the rose was seen as the symbol and provider of ageless beauty and research is proving that this idea isn't far off. As a known cicatrisant, rose essential oil affects the skin in a revolutionary way. While so many creams and lotions simply sit on the surface to the skin and provide temporary benefits, because of its natural structure, rose oil is well absorbed by the dermis and makes changes to the skin cells. This allows for cellular regeneration and new skin cells means that dull, dry, cracked and wrinkled skin is replaced with newer, firmer and younger looking skin. Rose oil is so good at this that it actually reduces the appearance and severity of lines, old scars and discoloration such as brown spots on the skin's surface. If you need to overhaul your complexion or treat a badly scarred, pocked or otherwise marked area of the skin, don't waste your time with over-the-counter scar remedies. Instead, regularly massage 3 drops of rose oil mixed with 1 tablespoon of coconut oil into the affected are 2-3 times a week. Within a month, you'll see noticeable improvement.

For its Ability to Fight Off Infectious Diseases: Imagine a substance so potent, it can keep life-threatening diseases such as cholera, typhoid and bacterial diarrhea away. Well, rose oil is precisely that substance and while its bacteria-killing properties show no mercy to infectious conditions, it cleanses, purifies and prevents while still remaining a safe and natural alternative to toxic germicidal sprays and soaps. In fact, you can make your own rose oil spray by diluting 7-8 drops of the oil in an ounce of pure water and using this mixture as a disinfectant around the house, office, gym or anywhere else you're likely to come into contact with bacteria. Spray this mixture onto door handles and surfaces and allow it to work for 3-5 minutes, before wiping off with a paper towel.

For its Ability to Kill off Fungi: Most anti-fungal preparations are unnecessarily harsh on the body while not working as thoroughly as desired against the actual fungal infection. Rose oil is just the opposite. Gentle on you but tough on fungi, this oil is a perfect antidote to candida, oral thrush and any other systemic, chronic and hard-to-treat fungal infections.

Aromatherapy: Because fungi can be removed from one part of the body, only to take cover in another part, use rose oil in the following all over, anti-fungal treatment, for best results: Combine 1 cup of pink Himalayan sea salt and 8 drops of rose oil in a warm bath. Soak from head to toe in the water for at least 15 minutes. Do this twice a week, for serious fungal relief. To obtain smooth, even-toned and ageless skin, add 2 drops of rose oil to a water moistened cotton ball and work over the face, jaw line and neck 3 to 4 times a week. You can also make an aromatic treatment by mixing 2 drop of rose oil with 1 drop of frankincense essential oil and diluting in an ounce of olive oil. Cleanse the skin thoroughly and then apply this blend by patting it into the skin.

Precautions to Remember: Rose oil is undoubtedly the queen of all essential oils. However, it's important to keep in mind that more than 11,000 rose petals must be used to make one small bottle of rose oil and this makes the oil very costly to produce. As a result, many of the so-called "rose oils" out there today actually contain less than 5 % of real rose oil. The rest of the mixture is made up of solvents or other inferior oils. Be careful when purchasing this oil and always look for companies that can guarantee the purity of their rose oil. This is very critical, as using impure oil in topical applications or baths could have negative health consequences. Pregnant and nursing women as well as young children should only use this oil under the guidance and advice of a doctor. Avoid allowing the oil into your eyes, nose, or ears. While rose oil is quite safe in its pure form, it can be expensive so make your bottle last longer by diluting with safe carrier oils in a rose oil to carrier ratio of 1to 3.

Chapter 17

S.

Sandalwood Oil:

Sandalwood oil is expressed from the heartwood of the East Indian sandalwood tree. This precious ancient essential oil has a history of over 4000 years of use and in modernity, it continues to be valued and employed for its many benefits.

For its Uniquely Healing Properties: Did you know that recent research has found that when your skin "smells" sandalwood oil, it actually begins to heal itself? It's true! Sandalwood oil activates scent receptors located throughout the body and on the skin in particular. When this happens, tests show that the skin begins to trigger a range of wound healing, collagen rebuilding and other rejuvenating activities.

For Treating Respiratory Conditions: Sandalwood oil is famed for its ability to clear out the throat, lungs and chest and support overall respiratory health. To access this healing, simply fill a large bowl with steaming water, mix in 5-6 drops of sandalwood oil and while making sure to stay about 10 inches away from the bowl, make a tent over your head and the bowl with a clean towel. This will trap the rising scented steam and allow you to breathe in all of the expectorant and cleansing properties. If you have a cold, throat or chest infection, do this every 2 days, to remove any infected phlegm and disinfect the area.

For its Soothing Components: Sandalwood oil is jam-packed with components that can clear up irritation and inflammation, so if you're raw, itchy or red, this oil is for you. Because inflammatory conditions are directly responsible for psoriasis, acne, eczema and other rashes, clearing up the source of the fire is the first step in clearing these reactions up. To get the benefits of this skin-soothing oil, mix 3 drops of sandalwood oil into 1 tablespoon of jojoba oil and apply to areas of irritation. This will calm even the reddest, roughest scales and return skin to its normal, healthy state.

For its Dermal Antiseptic Qualities: Not only is this oil great for reducing irritation but it can also be used to cleanse sin wounds and eruptions. If you're suffering from sores, boils, wounds or acne pustules, first cleanse the skin. Then, apply a thin layer of sandalwood oil, blended with coconut oil. As the anti-septic oil sinks into the skin, any infectious pathogens, unclean debris and other toxins will be removed from the irritated area. Regularly cleansing sores and pustules with sandalwood oil will result in quicker healing and lowers the risk of permanent scarring.

Many people who overuse antibiotics experience a depletion of good bacteria and an overgrowth of bad bacteria. This can often result in skin infections and lesions that are hard to get under control. Sandalwood oil works by using both its cleansing and anti-inflammatory qualities to destroy bad bacteria and calm down inflammation. Another great benefit of using this oil in such cases is that the components of sandalwood oil are tough on germs but not on your delicate complexion.

For its Deodorizing Properties: Sandalwood oil was one of the original deodorants and perfumes used in the ancient world. Today, it is still beloved for its ability to purify the skin, rebalance the sweat and impart a wonderful woody scent to the whole body. If you are leery of using commercial deodorizing preparations but still want to smell great, try making a blend of 2 drops of sandalwood oil in 1 tablespoon of olive oil and applying to the underarms and other areas where you sweat most often. Allow the blend to sit for at least half an hour before washing off and you'll find that sandalwood's antiseptic and anti-odor action leaves you smelling fresh all day.

For its Ability to Boost Cognitive Functions: Research has shown us that just smelling sandalwood oil can markedly improve an individual's ability to focus, think and remember , while also increasing relaxation. Unlike lavender oil, sandalwood relaxes and increases cognitive abilities, without making you sleepy. If you need an all-natural study air or a concentration boost at work, try diffusing a couple of drops of the oil at your desk, for a calming but fatigue-free way to help you achieve your work and studying goals.

For its Ability to Cure Bladder Infections: Those who have recurring bladder infections and can't get the relief they need with conventional medications rely on sandalwood oil. Adding 7-8 drops of the oil into a warm bath and soaking allows sandalwood's antiseptic, anti-pathogenic and inflammation cooling qualities to clear up any infections and restore the body to health. Even better, because it is a natural product, you don't have to worry about infections becoming resistant to treatment.

Aromatherapy: Place 3 drops of sandalwood oil in a nebulizer and inhale the vapors or try using it in a diffuser or oil lamp, for a long lasting, cognition-boosting scent. Sandalwood oil also works to improve high blood pressure, so regularly apply a couple of drops in olive oil, directly to the skin to gain a decrease in your blood pressure levels. Using sandalwood oil in a steam inhalation or a diffuser can both be excellent ways to treat respiratory infections, soothe coughs and asthma and decrease stress. Adding 5 -6 drops of sandalwood oil to your bath water at night can decrease insomnia.

Alternatively, you can place 2 drops of the oil on your pillow, for deep, peaceful sleep. Make sure that you place the drops on the side of the pillow you'll be sleeping on, so that you can inhale the calming fragrance all night. If you feel a sore throat coming on, simply add 2-3 drops of this oil into a glass of water and gargle thoroughly. The anti-bacterial and inflammation-fighting nature of sandalwood oil will heal your throat in not time.

Precautions to Remember: Sandalwood oil has been used for many centuries and as a result, we know it is a gentle, effective and generally safe substance. However, keep the following in mind for best results: Sandalwood oil can be consumed but should only be used orally under strict medical supervision. Photosensitivity may occur if skin treated with this oil is exposed to direct sunlight. It's important to always dilute sandalwood oil before applying. This oil can be diluted in a carrier oil, unscented lotion or even water. Pregnant and nursing women and very young children should not use sandalwood oil. If you have any preexisting health issues, please consult with your doctor before making sandalwood oil a regular part of your healthcare routine. While sandalwood oil is commonly used to calm anxious pets, certain pets may find the oil toxic so it is necessary to consult a veterinarian before using it on animals.

Chapter 18
T.

Thyme Essential Oil:

Thyme essential oil is a warmly aromatic and highly healing oil. It has historically been used to give relief to people suffering from a diverse array of conditions, from arthritis to stomach cramps, nerve disorders to infectious diseases. In aromatherapy, thyme oil's pleasing fragrance and concentrated properties have made it a firm favorite. Let's take a look at some of the qualities of this ancient essential oil:

For Hair Loss: One of thyme oils most well-known qualities is its ability to promote the growth of a healthy head of hair. Practitioners and aromatherapy enthusiasts have been using this oil for years to put a stop to sudden hair loss, prevent further hair loss and heal scalp conditions, making it possible to grow strong, thick hair. Thyme oil is so beneficial for hair growth and treating hair loss that it has even been called "nature's Rogaine!"

For Protection from Super Bugs: Today, modern medicine is struggling to cope with a serious threat to health- medicine resistant strains of virulent bacteria. These "super bugs" such as MRSA and others have become accustomed to all forms of conventional treatment, making them especially aggressive and hard to fight. That's where powerful essential oils like thyme come in. Thyme oil's naturally anti-septic, antimicrobial components, such as caryophyllene and camphene instantly attack and weaken these dangerous bacterial strains. When conventional medical treatments fail, using thyme oil can yield surprising results. In recent tests, thyme oil was found to be very effective at destroying many different types of Staphylococcus strains and doctors believe it may be a great alternative to powerful antibiotics!

For Spasms: This oil is also a potent antispasmodic substance. If you are dealing with any kind of painful, involuntary contraction or cramp, whether in the chest, stomach area or even the muscles, simply smelling thyme oil can help to quickly relieve the pain and cramping. Thyme oil has been found to be particularly useful in reducing menstrual cramps for women and also easing after-work out aches.

For Cardiac Disorders: Cardiac diseases are perhaps the greatest health threat facing us in modern times. That's why thyme oil's amazingly heart–protective effects are something to really pay attention to. It contributes to maintaining valve health and functionality, boosts the heart's strength and lowers rates of cardiac inflammation. As a relaxant, thyme oil also eases the tension in veins and arteries.

For Its Anti-Rheumatic Qualities: Thyme oil is an excellent, natural way to fight off rheumatism, gout and arthritic conditions throughout the body. These disorders occur either because the body is experiencing poor circulation or because uric acid and other toxins and impurities are not being fully and regularly eliminated from the system. As these toxins buildup in the blood, they contribute to inflammation and end up causing illness. Thyme oil is both a stimulating substance and a diuretic agent. As a stimulant, it improves blood circulation throughout the body and as a diuretic, it causes frequent urination, allowing built-up toxins to be drawn out of the body through waste byproducts. The result is that painful conditions like gout and arthritis are quickly and safely soothed and healed.

For Improper Water Elimination and Kidney Disorders: These days as our diets and our environments become increasingly loaded with pollutants and hard to handle chemicals, our body's natural waste elimination protocols are severely challenged. An inability to eliminate water from the body is the first sign that the body is having difficulty detoxifying itself. Symptoms such as swelling, bloating, heaviness and edema all point to the poor functioning of the kidneys. If nothing is done to support the kidneys, renal failure may occur. Luckily, using thyme oil in massages, inhalations and soaks offers us a wonderful way to offer the kidneys the help they need. Through its diuretic and cleansing qualities, this oil removes excess salts and water from the body, taking with it many harmful substances that the kidneys struggle to process. This deeply detoxifying effect makes thyme oil a valuable addition to any weight loss or blood pressure lowering health plan.

Aromatherapy:

You can gain the benefits of thyme essential oil in many different ways. Whether you inhale it, use it topically, or in soaks and cleansers, this oil can improve your health and appearance in ways that are truly noticeable.

Add 3-4 drops of thyme oil to a warm bath to get rid of exhaustion and soothes aches and spasms.

Blend 4 drops of thyme oil into 1 tablespoon of almond oil and massage any tender, sore or stiff areas with this oil mix, for fast pain relief.

Diffuse 2-3 drops of thyme oil throughout your bedroom, to access better, sounder sleep. You can also make a stronger diffusion of the oil, adding 4-5 drops and diffusing this antibacterial scent in areas that require disinfection.

Make a steam inhalation by adding 2-3 drops of thyme oil to a large bowl of hot water and creating a tent over your face with a clean cloth or towel. This oil's cleansing steam will remove infected mucus in the case of colds and flus and will relieve blocked or stuffed sinuses during allergy season.

Use thyme as a natural cleanser. Add 3 drops of thyme oil to your favorite unscented face wash and allow the mix to penetrate the pores for 5-8 minutes, before rinsing off for cleaner, acne-free skin. You can also use 2 drops of thyme in a cup of water for oral cleanliness. Swish this mixture around your mouth thoroughly, to banish germs, plaque and bad breath. This mouth wash will leave your mouth feeling and smelling fresh for longer than most commercially available mouth washes.

Precautions to Remember: As with all highly beneficial essential oils, thyme oil is very concentrated. Although its wonderful properties can offer a fast track to good health for most people, pregnant and nursing women, young children and those who are susceptible to high blood pressure should avoid using this oil.

Chapter 19

V.

Valerian Essential Oil

Valerian essential oil is produced from heavily scented and medicinal valerian flowers. With its ability to ease, soothe and relax a variety of conditions, valerian oil is known as "the calmer". You can use this oil:

For its Sleep Inducing Properties:

Valerian oil is one of nature's oldest cures for insomnia and sleep disorders. Long before the advent of modern day sleeping pills, people historically used this essential oil to create the perfect conditions for good quality sleep. This oil works by balancing hormonal levels within the body to promote deep, peaceful sleep.

For its Naturally Anti-Depressant Properties: Did you know that valerian essential oil is one of the most effective ways to treat depression and anxiety? Valerian is so effective in fact, that today's Valium drug is actually based on this amazing essential oil's qualities! In the same way that this oil rebalances delicate hormonal levels within the body to promote sleep, it also lowers levels of harmful stress hormones that contribute to depression and anxiety, creating a calming, relaxed and in-control feeling for those who use it. Reducing stress hormones also plays a part in overall health. High stress hormones contribute to weight gain, collagen depletion, memory loss and even long-term brain shrinkage! Valerian oil combats this by creating a peaceful sensation in the mind and harmonizing hormone levels in the body.

For its Ability to Boost Brain Power:

You can use valerian essential oil to give your brain a helpful boost. Because this essential oil actively affects and stimulates many different regions of the brain, it can result in better, sharper and faster thinking. It also allows users to understand more complex ideas and improves problem solving skills in regular users. Whether you're pulling an all-night study session or you fear your cognitive abilities are growing dull with time or fatigue, this oil is an amazing restorer of cognition. This brain stimulating ability makes valerian oil a great option for those who are seeking a good natural memory strengthener and can be used by elderly people, to significantly decrease the risk of developing Alzheimer's disease, various types of dementia and any other age-related cognitive diseases. To make the most of valerian's brain boosting properties, use an inhalation, as scent directly impacts he brain.

Heart Palpitations:

A rapid heart rate and heart palpitations can start to negatively affect your heart's condition, over time.

It's important to see a doctor about any heart conditions you may be suffering from, but with professional medical supervision, valerian essential oil can be used to calm and control the heart and regulate its actions. That's because medical research now backs up this oil's reputation as a cardiac calmer. Tests show that valerian oil's highly active components can ease an erratic heart rate, decrease heart palpitations and improve the heart's overall condition.

For its Hypotensive Effects:

 Internally consuming valerian essential oil can decrease high blood pressure levels, through the very same mechanisms that make this oil an amazing calmer of the heart rate and the emotions. While hypertension is a serious disorder requiring medical care, adding valerian oil to your health regimen can protect your from strokes, heart attacks and permanent cardiovascular damage.

Aromatherapy:

 Diffuse 2-3 drops of valerian oil at your desk, to improve your ability to work or study. If you're facing a test or a particularly tough meeting, take a sniff of the oil from its bottle, for a quick brain-sharpening boost. For mild depression, add 2 drops of the oil to your pillow or bedsheets until you see an improvement in mood. For cardiac protection and to lower blood pressure, consume the oil internally. Add 1-2 drops of valerian oil to a glass of pure water and drink this mix 2 or 3 times a week. To induce peaceful sleep, take a bath using 5-6 drops of the oil in warm water, about half an hour before bedtime.

Precautions to Remember:

As long as you consume it in very low doses, valerian essential oil is widely believed to be quite safe for internal use. This potent oil's effects will be felt at even the smallest doses, so resist the urge to add more than a drop or two to your glass of water. Pregnant and nursing women, people with preexisting health conditions and small children should never use valerian oil in any form without medical supervision or advice. Ingesting too much of this oil can lead to cramps, loss of orientation, fatigue and even allergic rashes. These effects are rare and can usually be avoided through proper dosing.

Chapter 20

W.

White Fir Essential Oil:

Essential oil expressed from the white fir tree is an alpine, woodsy smelling and deeply refreshing substance that has become a pain-killing favorite for aromatherapy enthusiasts. Unlike many other essential oils, white fir oil has a crisp, fresh and masculine scent that revitalizes the senses. Here are some fantastic applications for this rare oil:

For Joint and Muscle Health:

Many people who make a career out of movement, such as competitive athletes and performers, have long used white fir oil for the joint protective and pain easing benefits it offers. Simply massaging the diluted oil into the skin can drastically increase flexibility and mobility, while using it before workouts or heavy physical activity can result in less strains, pulls and soreness. The next time you have a swollen, stiff joint or are experiencing deep muscular pain anywhere in your body, try reaching for white fir oil instead of for an over-the-counter painkiller. You'll be amazed by how quickly and completely this cooling oil banishes pain!

For its Ability to Cleanse, Heal and Support the Respiratory System: This particular benefit makes white fir oil a must-have during the colder months or in flu and hay fever seasons. The refreshing nature of this oil helps it to open up blocked, congested airways, making breathing easier. It can also be used to disinfect the respiratory system, through inhalation and diffusing and can help to remove excess mucus through its role as a mild expectorant.

For its Dermal Soothing Qualities: As with all tree oils, white fir essential oil provides dry, rough and irritated skin with a soothing, calming remedy. If your skin suffers from cracking, weeping and stretching during the winter months, try a warm, but not overly hot, bath using white fir oil. Its skin healing abilities will have your skin feeling and looking brand new again, in no time. This oil is also great for burning, itching scalp so you can either add a couple of drops to your shampoo or simply allow your head to soak in a mixture of 1 cup water and 4-5 drops of white fir oil. Massaging this mixture into the scalp will help the healing to begin even faster.

Aromatherapy:

Use white fir essential oil to soothe away joint and muscle aches and pains by adding 7-8 drops of the oil to a warm and relaxing bath. You can also choose to make an effective pain-killing rub by mixing 3-4 drops of white fir oil into a tablespoon of olive oil and massaging any painful areas thoroughly. If you are suffering from breathing difficulties or want to fight off an encroaching cold or flu, simply diffuse 2-3 drops of the oil in a diffuser and inhale the cleansing, strengthening scent. If you are already in the midst of a respiratory infection, applying an oil blend made of 3-4 drops of white fir oil and one and a half tablespoons of olive oil to the chest and upper back areas can help you to open up the lungs and remove infected phlegm. If you need to quickly fight off fatigue, place 2 drops of white fir oil on the soles of your feet and massage deeply.

Precautions to Remember:

Because some people have heightened sensitivities to tree oils, remember to do a patch test before using this oil. Testing your reaction to a small application on the feet is a good way to gauge your tolerance level. Using this or any other oil excessively could result in skin sensitization. Do not use this oil in the eyes, nose or mouth area. Seek medical advice before using this oil on pregnant and nursing women as well as young children.

Chapter 21
Y.

<u>Ylang Ylang Essential Oil:</u>

Ylang ylang essential oil (*Cananga odorata*) is an exotic, sweet smelling, floral oil produced from the South East Asian ylang ylang flower. Far from being just a lavishly fragrant substance, this oil can provide healing, calming and balancing for the body and mind.

For its Overall Body Balancing Properties:
Ylang ylang essential oil provides far-reaching benefits for the body's hormonal production system, the endocrine system and the cardiovascular system. Just the scent of ylang ylang alone can set off a cycle of events that promote hormonal rebalancing and result in more energy and better health.

In fact, in several studies, those who inhaled this essential oil's scent were found to have much lower levels of the stress hormone cortisol, as a result. If you are under a heavy workload or facing other sources of stress and anxiety, using ylang ylang oil in an inhalation or diffusion can help to alleviate the effects of tension, by reducing the levels of cortisol-led damage you may sustain.

For its Relaxation Inducing Effects:

Ylang ylang essential oil has proved to effectively reduce stress levels in those who inhale it or apply it to skin. This oil provides a strong but completely natural anxiety-lowering and antidepressant-like effect on the mind. In one study, 24 healthy people were exposed to the scent of ylang ylang essential oil. This resulted in a rapid lowering of their pulse rates and blood pressure levels. The oil also appeared to increase their calm, focus and alertness.

For its Skin and Hair Nourishing Qualities:

Nothing moisturizes, restores and replenishes dry skin like ylang ylang oil. With over 165 active components, this oil quickly and deeply enters the dermis to create fuller, firmer and less wrinkled skin. When used on dry, flaky and itchy areas, it can reduce irritation, calm inflammation, promote healing of any wounds and restore the balance of moisture in parched skin.

When massaged regularly into the scalp, ylang ylang oil is an efficient alopecia-fighting substance. It's previously mentioned ability to balance hormone levels contributes to the regrowth of healthy hair.

Aromatherapy:

There are many ways to garner the positive rewards of ylang ylang essential oil use. To aid in full body relaxation, place 7-8 drops of the oil into a bath, along with Epsom salts and soak for 15-20 minutes.

For smooth, blemish-free and rejuvenated skin, add 4-5 drops of ylang ylang oil to a bowl of steaming water and give yourself an aromatherapy facial. Massage a blend of 2 tablespoons of jojoba oil and 4 drops of ylang ylang oil into any tense areas, such as the jaws, shoulders and upper back, This will loosen the tension while also allowing ylang ylang to exert a positive effect on the hormonal system. Place 2-3 drops of the oil into your favorite conditioner and add 1 tablespoon of coconut oi. Massage this mixture into the hair and allow it to sit for 5-10 minutes, for smooth, silky and vibrant hair.

Precautions to Remember: Ylang ylang oil has very few reported side effects and is often thought to be the mildest and one of the safest oils to use. If you are prone to sensitivities however, always test ylang ylang essential oil on a small area of the skin before using it in larger applications, in order to avoid an allergic reaction. If possible, it is best to begin usage by applying a small amount of the oil to the feet and progressing from there, if there are no reactions. Avoid using this and all other essential oils excessively, in order to avoid sensitization and irritation of the skin. Make sure to keep the oil out of your nose, eyes and ears.

As using ylang ylang oil internally could result in toxicity, I don't recommend that you consume this oil. Instead, make sure to use it in topical applications, diluted with carrier oils such as jojoba, coconut, olive or almond oil or in diffusions.

Pregnant and nursing women should consult a doctor before using this and all other essential oils. It's also best to seek medical advice before using ylang ylang oil on young children. Be careful to use ylang ylang oil according to the instructions on the bottle and when in doubt, consult a trained aromatherapy professional.

Chapter 22:

Z.

Zataria Essential Oil:

Zataria essential oil is expressed from the plant *Zataria mulitiflora,* also widely known as thyme of Shiraz. This flowering herb grows mainly in South West Asia and its essential oil has been traditionally used for centuries as an intensely healing, restorative and tonic substance. It has well-known uses as a carminative, antiseptic, stimulant, anesthetic diaphoretic, and diuretic oil. It is also a useful anti-spasmodic and often employed as a powerful natural painkiller. Let's look at some of the best ways to use this rare and precious essential oil:

For its Antimicrobial Powers:

Zataria oil can be used as an extremely effective antimicrobial treatment. This oil contains many highly active compounds that destroy and completely eradicate many tough-to-treat bacteria strains. Two of its most potent components are thymol and carvacol. These oxygenated monoterpenes are behind Zataria oil's reputation as a cleansing, purifying wound healing and anti-infection oil. It works to disrupt the growth of several harmful pathogenic infectious agents such as *Klebsiella*, *E.coli* and *Staphylococcus aureus* and is effective against both Gram-positive and Gram-negative bacteria types.

To use this oil against infections of the biliary tract, the urinary tract or to discourage infectious growth in wounds, diffuse a couple of drops and inhale the scent. Alternatively, you can inhale the oil directly from the bottle or apply in a diluted form, with carrier oils, to areas of skin that require anti-infection support. Zataria oil is particularly good to diffuse or use in steam inhalations after a surgical operation, to cleanse and heal wounds quickly. Before using the oil in this application, always consult with your doctor first.

This oil is also an established anti-fungal treatment option and has been proven to work against candida as well as *Malassezia* fungal infections.

For Its Ability to Fight Off H. Pylori Infections:

H. pylori is an extremely aggressive and difficult to eradicate stomach bug that is now known to be the primary cause of stomach ulcers. This type of bacteria is behind the widespread prevalence of symptoms such as indigestion, nausea, flatulence and gastric reflux.

It is thought to affect up to 50% of the population and can lurk secretly inside the stomach for many years, causing silent but serious damage. Recently, many antibiotics have become totally ineffective against H. pylori. Fortunately, researchers have now proved that Zataria essential oil is an excellent treatment alternative. Due to the oil's high carvacol content, it appears to quickly and thoroughly weaken and wipe out H. pylori colonies and is much gentler on the already damaged stomach lining than most conventional medications. Best of all, ingestion is not necessary and bacteria elimination occurs even after using the oil in a simple inhalation.

Aromatherapy:

Place 2-3 drops of Zataria essential oil on a diffuser and allow the scent to waft around, in order to disinfect rooms. Mix 3-4 drops of the oil in half an ounce of warm water and use this liquid to gargle away any sore throats or oral infections. Blend 3-4 drops of the oil to a tablespoon of olive or almond oil and apply this mixture to areas of skin that are infected or inflamed. You can also use this blend on wounds, to speed up healing and discourage bacterial infections. For fungal infections of the feet or nails, apply 4-5 drops of Zataria oil in one tablespoon of olive oil and allow the oil to sit for at least half an hour, before washing with warm water. For internal infections, you can fill a bathtub with warm water and mix in 8-9 drops of the oil. As you soak, make a point of inhaling the fragrant steam. This will allow the antibacterial scent to work its way into the respiratory system, while the water and oil solution soaks into the skin.

Precautions to Remember:

As with all potent essential oils, pregnant and nursing women as well as individuals with preexisting conditions should all consult with a doctor before using this oil. As the oil is very concentrated, do not use on very young children unless directed to do so by a health professional. Because Zataria oil tends to be rare, it is important to make sure that the bottle of oil you are using is pure and does not contain any chemical additive s or fillers. Do not use on eyes, ears or nose. Before attempting to consume Zataria essential oil, speak with your doctor or a professional aromatherapy specialist, to find out if this method of treatment is right for you.

Chapter 23:

A Last Word on Using Oils Wisely:

By now, you know just how powerfully healing essential oils can be. But it is important to keep in mind that all of this power comes with a caveat. Safety must always come first when using these oils, because healing can only occur when harm is avoided. That's why I wanted to include additional safety guidelines, to help you navigate through the world of aromatherapy safely, effectively and problem-free. However, please do not take these rules as definitive. Because each person is different and preexisting health conditions can and do affect the way these oils work, I recommend that you always speak to a doctor or homeopathic medical practitioner about any questions or concerns you may have. With that said, these guidelines below are a great starting point and will help to see you through the initial stages of your healing journey.

Consider this: Essential oils are far more concentrated than most people realize. Consider this: On average, it takes literally hundreds of pounds of flowers or plants to make just one pound of essential oil! That's why essential oils provide a highly magnified version of benefits, but that's also why we must be very careful when using them. Just because they are derived from natural sources does not mean that we can simply use and misuse them as we wish In fact, because nature often provides the most powerful substances, we sometimes have to be even more careful when using nature-based products like essential oils, than we would be with weaker, synthetic products.

Always Dilute: I cannot stress this enough. Essential oils often come in small bottles because just one drop contains more potent compounds than several ounces or even cups of any other substance. While there may be exceptions, I generally advise very strongly against using an essential oil on the skin in undiluted form. These oils are extremely biologically active and will wind up in the bloodstream much faster than you may imagine. Thus, you should always use a stable carrier oil such as olive oil, jojoba oil or coconut oil, to cut the strength of these essential oils. Another bonus is that, when you use carrier oils, you are stretching out those sometimes expensive bottles of essential oils and making your aromatherapy regimen more efficient AND more effective.

 Test Yourself: I personally recommend doing a simple patch test before using any new essential oil for the first time. Dilute the new oil and apply a small amount of it to the feet. After observing the area, if you don't notice any irritation or discoloration within 24 hours, you can go ahead and try using the oil on a larger area.

Do Not Use On Pregnant or Nursing Women and on Babies or Young Children: These guidelines are hands down, the most important ones to pay attention to. That's because due to a variety of different reasons, essential oils are way too strong to be used in such cases. When in doubt, always consult a doctor first. Still, you can't go wrong by avoiding essential oils during the sensitive stages of pregnancy, breastfeeding and early childhood.

Photosensitivity:

Many oils can cause photosensitivity, leading to painful irritation of the skin, eruption of blister, discoloration, scarring and even fever-like conditions. This occurs when skin treated with photosensitivity-causing oil is exposed to the sun within 24 hours of oil application. While a large number of oils can cause photosensitivity, the most common offenders are citrus oils such as lemon, lime, grapefruit, orange and bergamot oil.

Consuming Essential Oils: It is important to note that many oils should NOT be consumed due to toxicity, extreme concentration or unsuitability for the human gut. While consuming certain oils may leave you feeling sick, taking others internally could actually be life-threatening. Remember that most essential oils are as strong as dozens and sometimes hundreds of cups of herbal tea and that each little bottle contains many, many pounds of the source plant within it. Only use oil's according to instructions, and again, when in doubt, ask a doctor or homeopathic health practitioner. When you do consume an oil, please do so under medical supervision or advice, to be absolutely safe.

Only Use Pure, Organic and Good Quality Oils: As essential oils are ultra-concentrated, it's extremely important to make sure that you are not putting any toxic or sub-par imitations into your body. Only use oil's from reputable suppliers and always make sure that the oils are free from any chemical additives. Know what is really in the bottle before you risk putting it in your delicate system. Many unscrupulous essential oil sellers provide mixes, in which the pure oil is blended with synthetic fragrances, solvents and other highly poisonous items. Needless to say, such oils are a real health hazard and should not be used. Also, never purchase an oil in a plastic bottle. Essential oils are so powerful that they eventually eat through plastic and should only be stored in glass bottles.

And The Last Rule of Essential Oils….Enjoy!

This isn't really a rule, but rather a reminder. While there are some guidelines to keep in mind, essential oils are extremely potent, effective, safe, fragrant and pleasant. They provide healing, balance the body and mind and can significantly improve your well-being, your fitness and even your appearance. As you go further in your aromatherapy journey, remember that you can use this guide to easily access all of the information you need to make the best decisions for your wellness. Simply use the alphabetized format to flip to the oil you want to learn more about and you'll quickly find all of the benefits, methods of use and safety information for your oil of choice, at your fingertips. In closing, I'd like to thank you for accompanying me on this discovery of the wonderfully renewing, health-promoting world of essential oils and aromatherapy.

Essential oils bring the thousands of healing plant and flower components that humanity has relied on for millennia to you. These components will literally change your life with their intense restorative powers and will help you to depend less and less on the harsh medications and invasive treatments of conventional medicine. There is absolutely no part of your physical or mental health that cannot be improved, restored or transformed by using essential oils and aromatherapy techniques. Make sure to flip to the bonus index of powerful recipes and blends at the end of this chapter, for natural and potent remedies that you can use year in and year out.

Use this guide and all of the oils contained in it, wisely and well and may you enjoy them in good physical and mental health!

****
****

___Recipe Index: Amazing and Easy Ways to Use Aromatherapy For Healing and Weight Loss___

Now that you know the properties, powers and safety information of these essential oils, it's time to have some fun with mixing, blending and creating your very own aromatherapy diffuser formulas for every ailment under the sun. Enjoy!

For Weight Loss:

To maintain balanced blood sugar and reduce carbohydrate and sugar cravings, simply diffuse a blend of 3 drops of grapefruit oil and 4 drops of cinnamon oil. Inhale the scent deeply.

Give yourself the energy you need for workouts by blending 3 drops each of bergamot oil and grapefruit oil.

Make a diffusion of 4 drops of clove oil and 2 drops of cinnamon oil to speed up your metabolism and help control your appetite.

For Energy and Revitalization:

- Mix 4 drops of peppermint oil and 4 drops of grapefruit oil and diffuse this blend to rev up your energy levels.
- Blend 4 drops of lemon oil, 4 drops of grapefruit oil and 2 drops of lavender oil and diffuse to achieve alertness.
- Blend 3 drops each of Frankincense, basil and ginger oil and add to your diffuser, for a clear mind and a wide awake sensation.

For Anti-Anxiety and Antidepressant Effects:

- Diffuse 2 drops of lavender oil, 2 drops of bay oil and 4 drops of bergamot oil to achieve relaxation and keep feel-good hormones flowing.
- Make a citrus-sensation diffusion by blending cheerful oils such as 3 drops of orange oil, 3 drops of grapefruit oil and 3 drops of lemon oil.
- To do away with the winter weather blues, blend 3 drops of cinnamon oil, 2 drops of

bergamot oil and 2 drops of sandalwood and add to your diffuser.

For Anti-Insect Action:

- Blend and diffuse 3 drops of eucalyptus oil and 3 drops of thyme oil, to ward off mosquitoes.
- Get rid of flying and crawling pests around the home by mixing and diffusing 4 drops of peppermint oil, 3 drops of bergamot oil and 3 drops of eucalyptus oil.
- For a quick cleansing way to keep all bugs away try diffusing 5-6 drops of pure eucalyptus and 2 drops of lemon oil.

For Immune System Support:

- Keep your immune system strong all through winter by diffusing 2 drops of rosemary oil and 3 drops of clove oil.
- Blend 2 drops of orange oil, 2 drops of Douglas fir oil and 2 drops of oregano oil to disinfect areas and keep the flu at bay.
- Maintain a healthy respiratory system by diffusing 4 drops of frankincense oil and 2 drops of eucalyptus oil and inhaling the scent deeply.
- Combat allergies and blocked sinuses by making a blend of 2-3 drops of thyme oil, 5

drops of thyme oil and 3 drops of peppermint oil and diffuse.

- A diffusion of 4 drops lavender, 3 drops eucalyptus and 4 drops of bay oil will keep viruses and respiratory infections from gaining a foothold in your body.

For Digestive Health:

- Mix 4 drops of bay oil and 4 drops of dill seed oil. Diffuse this blend for an instant remedy to nausea and indigestion.
- Blend 3 drops of fennel oil and 2 drops of peppermint. Inhale this diffusion for a lighter feeling in the stomach and to stimulate a lost appetite.

For A Brain Boosting Session:

- Get your gray matter working smoothly by reducing inflammation with dill seed oil and angelica oil. Diffuse 4 drops of dill seed oil and 4 drops of angelica oil at your desk to stay on top of your cognitive game.
- Make an anti-inflammatory, brain-sharpening diffusion by mixing 6 drops of eucalyptus oil and 3 drops of bay oil.

****
****

<u>Definitive Tips for Using Essential Oil's For Weight Loss</u>

Grapefruit Oil:

To achieve rapid weight loss and support your diet and exercise regimen, try using these methods:

- Make a zingy fresh morning fat-burning beverage by mixing 1-2 drops of pure grapefruit oil in your glass of water. This will help you shed pounds and maintain high energy throughout the day.
- Inhale the scent of grapefruit oil straight from the bottle a few times a day, to keep your metabolism charged.
- Regularly rub areas where fat has accumulated or tough to lose fatty areas and cellulite with a blend of 3-4 drops of grapefruit oil in 1 ounce of extra virgin olive oil.

Bergamot Essential Oil:

To banish stress-eating and promote weight loss, try these tips:

- Massage the soles of your feet several times a week with a blend of 3-4 drops of bergamot oil in an ounce of coconut oil, to get rid of nervous-eating and improve your mood.
- Soak in a warm bath of 7 drops of bergamot oil and warm water. This will help reduce inflammatory conditions and promote fat-loss.

Sandalwood Oil:

This calming oil can relax the body and mind and in the process, gets rid of mindless eating and depression-related weight gain. Consider these methods:

- Rub 3-4 drops of sandalwood and an ounce of jojoba oil directly onto the stomach, the thighs and any other fatty areas.
- Inhale the scent of sandalwood in a diffusion or simply place 2 drops on a clean cloth and sniff throughout the day, to calm yourself and change bad eating habits.

Orange Oil:

This essential oil will help you make the most of your diet by reducing cravings, increasing fat-burning and keeping your metabolism high all day. Try the following:

- Use orange oil in diffusions throughout the home, kitchen and at your desk, wherever you need support to stop snacking. The citrusy scent will keep your hunger in check.
- Soak in an orange oil bath by adding 7 drops of it to warm water. This will work to reduce inflammation and cravings, while speeding up your metabolism.

Cinnamon Oil:

Use this sweetly spiced oil to gain powerful weight loss benefits in these ways:

- Start your day with one drop of cinnamon oil in a glass of water. This will start you off on the right foot and reduce hunger, while balancing blood sugar.
- For a quick way to improve insulin sensitivity, sniff 2-3 drops of cinnamon oil on a clean cloth.

- Make a truly fat melting massage oil out of a blend of 4 drops of cinnamon oil and an ounce of almond oil. Use this oil in full body massages, up to 3 times a week, for best results.

****

****

www.ingramcontent.com/pod-product-compliance
Lightning Source LLC
Chambersburg PA
CBHW071155280526
45787CB00002B/512